► ► ► ► • **Ethics in Medical Research:** A Handbook of Good Practice

All biomedical research proposals involving human subjects must be examined and approved by a research ethics committee or institutional review board. This ethical regulation can cause considerable delay to a research project, often simply because the ethical implications have not been considered.

This is a comprehensive and practical guide to the ethical issues raised by different kinds of medical research, and is the first such book to be written with the needs of researchers in mind. Clearly structured and written in a plain and accessible style, the book covers every significant ethical issue likely to be faced by researchers and research ethics committees. The author outlines and clarifies official guidelines, gives practical advice on how to adhere to these, and suggests procedures in areas where official recommendations are vague or absent.

This invaluable handbook will help researchers identify and address the ethical issues at an early stage in the design of their studies, to avoid unnecessary delay and to safeguard the well-being of patients and healthy volunteers. It will also be extremely useful to members of research ethics committees.

TREVOR SMITH is former scientific advisor to the Tayside Committee on Medical Research Ethics, and honorary lecturer in Epidemiology and Public Health Medicine at the University of Dundee. He has extensive experience as both a biomedical researcher and a research ethics committee member.

Ethics in Medical Research

A Handbook of Good Practice

Trevor Smith

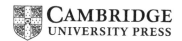

CAMBRIDGE
UNIVERSITY PRESS

PUBLISHED BY THE PRESS SYNDICATE OF THE UNIVERSITY OF CAMBRIDGE
The Pitt Building, Trumpington Street, Cambridge CB2 1RP, United Kingdom

CAMBRIDGE UNIVERSITY PRESS
The Edinburgh Building, Cambridge CB2 2RU, UK http://www.cup.cam.ac.uk
40 West 20th Street, New York, NY 10011-4211, USA http://www.cup.org
10 Stamford Road, Oakleigh, Melbourne 3166, Australia

First published 1999

Printed in the United Kingdom at the University Press, Cambridge

Typeset in Swift 9.25/13.5pt, in QuarkXPress™ [SE]

A catalogue record for this book is available from the British Library

Library of Congress Cataloguing in Publication data

Smith, Trevor, 1949- .
Ethics in medical research : a handbook of good practice / Trevor
Smith.
     p.   cm.
Includes bibliographical references and index.
ISBN 0 521 62619 6 (pbk.)
1. Human experimentation in medicine – Moral and ethical aspects.
2. Medicine – Research – Moral and ethical aspects.   I. Title.
[DNLM: 1. Ethics, Medical.   2. Research – organization &
administration.   3. Human Experimentation.   W 50s662e 1998]
R853.H8S64   1998
174'.28-dc21
DNLM/DLC   98-36842   CIP
for Library of Congress

ISBN 0 521 62619 6 paperback

The book is intended to alert researchers and others to the ethical issues raised by
different kinds of research, and should not be seen as a definitive statement of what can
or cannot be done. It is the ultimate responsibility of the researcher, his or her employer
and the local ethics committee to ensure that their research is always conducted to high
ethical standards and with due regard to the laws of the countries concerned.

This book is dedicated to

my parents, my wife Janette, and son David.

► Contents

▶ Preface

The amount of basic medical research and clinical trials conducted with patients and healthy volunteers continues to increase, with millions of people submitting themselves each year to extra procedures and new treatments in the hope of benefiting either themselves or patients in the future. But how well are their interests protected? Are researchers adequately equipped to tackle the increasingly complex ethical issues raised by different kinds of research old and new?

The World Medical Association's Declaration of Helsinki, the internationally accepted set of rules governing the conduct of medical research, requires that patients and healthy volunteers are fully informed about the research project and give written consent before they participate, but how well are the terms of the Declaration adhered to? Are prospective participants given enough time to decide whether to join a study and do they realise that participation is entirely voluntary and that they can withdraw at any time without giving a reason, or do they feel pressurised to participate, and if so, by who or by what?

A system of local medical research ethics committees or institutional review boards, designed to protect the interests of research participants by reviewing all proposals for research with people before they go ahead, is now being developed, or is already in operation, in most developed countries. How are such committees formed, who sits on them, what are their duties and how effective are they? How are the risks and benefits evaluated before patients are entered into a study? Is it ethical to use placebos in a clinical trial? Is it ever acceptable to conduct research with young children and others unable to give informed consent or to do research on people without their knowledge?

While new scientific developments, such as gene therapy, cloning and animal to human transplantation, will be expected to raise innumerable important ethical issues, even investigators making use of spare blood and other tissue samples need to be cautious. Suffice it to mention that hair clippings can be used to estimate past drug misuse, a placenta for developing agents of abortion and spare blood samples for testing for inherited late onset diseases, with profound implications for patients and their relatives. Even questionnaire studies are not always as innocent as they may seem, some questions being so tactless or intrusive as to cause severe alarm or distress. Studies that involve no more than access to patients' medical records, still raise important issues of confidentiality.

Should the responsibility of an ethics committee end with the approval of a study, or is there a case for committees to conduct on-site post approval review to ensure that the protocol they approved, and any conditions they imposed, are being adhered to? The final chapter is devoted to a discussion of its feasibility and value based on the experiences of the local Tayside Committee on Medical Research Ethics in undertaking post approval review.

This book is essentially a practical guide to help researchers to identify and address, at an early stage in the design of their studies, the ethical issues likely to be raised. In this way, it is hoped to avoid unnecessary delays to potentially valuable research. While national regulations and guidelines may differ in detail, the ethical issues raised by medical research remain the same, with researchers worldwide needing to conform to the Declaration of Helsinki.

Although this book has been primarily written for researchers and members of ethics committees, it is hoped that it will also be of value both to current and to potential participants. It should form a useful addition to the libraries of the many patient self-help groups springing up in towns and villages throughout the world that provide advice and comfort for patients with a wide variety of conditions. Many of these groups serve patients with conditions such as asthma, diabetes and psoriasis, who are in high demand as research subjects, finding themselves being invited to participate in yet another project almost every time they visit their family doctor or outpatient clinic. Also discussed are the ground rules of medical research, what the patients' rights are and how they should expect to be treated, which hopefully will help strengthen the partnership between patient and researcher to the benefit of both. Last, but by no means least, this book should also be of value to academic ethicists and students with an interest in practical medical ethics.

► Acknowledgements

For the wealth of ideas generated during discussions of the ethical issues raised by over a thousand individual research proposals, I thank ethics committee members past and present: Mr Jack Bowman, Dr Stella Clark, Dr W. F. Morrison Dorward, Dr J. Stuart Fair, Professor George A. Fenton, Mrs Sheila M. Findlay, Mr Malcolm J. Finlayson (Secretary), Mr Nigel G. E. Harris, Dr William Henney, Miss Elizabeth Macallan, Mr A. MacConnachie, Professor Marion E. T. McMurdo, Dr Eddie J. H. Moore, Dr Andrew Reid, Dr Mike Roworth, Mr Harry D. Sheldon, Professor Allan D. Struthers, Professor Hugh Tunstall-Pedoe, Dr David Walsh, Professor Ian D. Willock, Dr Phyllis M. Windsor.

Most grateful thanks also to the following researchers whose detailed discussions of their projects contributed so much to our understanding of the ethical issues encountered by researchers in the conduct of their research: Dr Imran Aziz, Professor Jill J. F. Belch, Dr Clare Bonner, Dr David T. Bowen, Dr Kieran C. Breen, Dr Christine Brierley, Dr Philip G. Cachia, Dr Sandra Carlyle, Dr John Cater, Dr Patrick F. W. Chien, Mrs Shona Colville, Dr Duncan L. W. Davidson, Dr Julian Davis, Dr Robert Dawe, Dr John Ellis, Dr Dafydd Evans, Dr Michael Faed, Dr James Ferguson, Dr Angela Gilbert, Dr D. Goudie, Miss Leslie Grant, Dr Alison Grove, Dr Janesh K. Gupta, Dr Moyra Guthrie, Dr David K. Harrison, Professor Peter W. Howie, Dr Harriet Hudson, Dr Robert Hume, Dr David Keily, Dr Faisel Khan, Dr Alastair G. McDiarmid, Professor John McEwen, Dr Ronald S. MacWalter, Dr Mohamed A. Mahgoub, Dr Pauline Maillou, Mr Mathews, Dr Gary Mires, Dr Ronald G. Neville, Dr G. R. Ogden, Professor Martin

Pippard, Dr Andrej T. Prach, Dr Gillian Pritchard, Dr Thomas Pullar, Dr Susan Rae, Dr Arthur Ratcliff, Dr Richard C. Roberts, Mrs Hazel Robertson, Dr Stuart T. D. Roxburgh, Dr Robin Smith, Dr Robert J. Swingler, Dr Ian Tait; Dr Kia Soong Tan, Dr Peter Thornton, Dr John Vernon, Dr John Winter, Mrs Janet Winter, Dr A. J. Wright.

Responsibility for the content of the book is, however, entirely mine.

The Declaration of Helsinki is reproduced with kind permission of the World Medical Association, the *Guideline for Good Clinical Practice* is reproduced with kind permission of the IFPMA, International Conference on Harmonisation and the list of research activities which may be reviewed through expedited review procedures is reproduced with kind permission of the Office for Protection from Research Risks, National Institutes of Health.

1

Origin of the ethical review of medical research

In past centuries we relied mainly on the integrity of the doctors concerned to decide whether the potential benefits to future patients and to society as a whole justified asking their patients and healthy volunteers to bear the risks of their research. Nowadays, patients are less likely to accept the old idea that the doctor is always right. Instead, they demand the autonomy to decide for themselves what procedures they are prepared to agree to and what treatments they are willing to receive.

It is likely that this trend would eventually have led to the regulation of experiments on humans, but it was the realisation of the appalling experiments that were carried out by groups of Nazi doctors during the Second World War which led to the first internationally recognised code of medical research ethics. This code, laid down in the course of a judgement during the Nuremberg War Crimes Trials, came to be known as the Nuremberg Code. It (Nuremberg Code 1946) sets 10 principles to which physicians must conform when conducting experiments on humans. The first of these principles stresses the need for voluntary informed consent. It defines informed consent and places responsibility for obtaining informed consent on the researcher. Other requirements include: experiments should not be random or unnecessary; experiments on humans should be preceded by experiments on animals and surveys of the natural history of the disease; unnecessary physical and mental suffering should be avoided; studies should be conducted by scientifically qualified professionals; subjects should be allowed to withdraw at any time; and investigators should be prepared to stop the research if at any time it appears that the subject is in danger.

The principles of this Code were incorporated by the medical profession in the Declaration of Helsinki, drawn up by the World Medical Association in 1964. The latest version of the Declaration (World Medical Association 1996) was approved at the 48th General Assembly of the World Medical Association held in the Republic of South Africa in 1996.

The Declaration of Helsinki

The 12 basic principles of the Declaration of Helsinki on biomedical research involving humans, with amendments, are summarised below:

(1) Biomedical research on human subjects must conform to accepted scientific principles.

(2) The design and performance of experimental procedures should be formulated in an experimental protocol and *approved by an ethics committee* independent of the investigator and the sponsor.

(3) The research should be conducted by scientifically qualified persons supervised by a medical clinician.

(4) The importance of the objective must be in proportion to the inherent risk to the subject.

(5) The research should be preceded by careful assessment of predictable risks. Concern for the interests of the subject must always prevail over the interests of science and society.

(6) Efforts must be made to minimise the impact on, and to respect, the subject's physical and mental integrity and privacy.

(7) Physicians must be satisfied that hazards are predictable and must stop if they outweigh benefits.

(8) Publications must be accurate and conform to these principles.

(9) Potential subjects must be informed of the aims, methods, anticipated benefits and potential hazards and discomforts

entailed and their right to abstain, or withdraw after giving consent.

(10) The physician must exercise particular care in obtaining consent from dependent subjects.

(11) Special consideration is necessary in the case of minors and others unable to give legal consent. Where a child is able to give consent, that consent, as well as that of the guardian should be obtained.

(12) The research protocol should contain a statement on the ethics and compliance with this Declaration.

Comments

The need for a written protocol that can be examined by an independent ethics committee should be recognised by all researchers. The protocol should be explicit as to what the research involves for the patients or healthy volunteers who are participating. If the proposal is approved and implemented, the written protocol must be followed. Any significant deviations from the protocol that have implications for the participants must be approved by the ethics committee before being implemented.

The Declaration draws a distinction between therapeutic research, where a treatment is being tested on patients, and non-therapeutic research aimed at gaining a better understanding of the nature of a disease and its causes.

Medical research combined with professional care (clinical research)

▶ The physician must be free to use new techniques if they offer hope of being beneficial.

▶ The potential hazards and discomforts of a new method must be balanced against those associated with the best current methods.

▶ Every patient, including controls, must be assured of the best proven diagnosis and therapy. (The following statement first appeared in the October 1996 Amendment.) This does not exclude the use of an inert placebo where no proven diagnostic or therapeutic method exists.

► Refusal to participate must never interfere with the physician–patient relationship.

► Any reasons for not obtaining informed consent must be incorporated in the research protocol for consideration by an *independent committee*.

► Research and medical care can be combined only to the extent that it is justified by its potential value to the patient.

Non-therapeutic biomedical research involving human subjects

► The physician must be the protector of the life and health of the experimental subject.

► Subjects must be volunteers – either healthy persons or patients.

► Research must be discontinued if continuation would be harmful to the subject.

► The interest of science and society should never take precedence over considerations related to the well-being of the subject.

The full text of the Declaration of Helsinki is reproduced in Appendix 1.

The evolution of ethics committees

The Nuremberg Code and the original Declaration of Helsinki (June 1964) did not refer to scrutiny by an independent ethics committee. This requirement arose with amendments made at the 29th General Assembly of the World Medical Association in Tokyo, Japan, in October 1975.

United States of America

In the USA, a number of key events can be identified that led to the setting up of ethics committees, as now required by the amended Declaration of Helsinki (World Medical Association 1996).

In 1953, the National Institutes of Health, at its new clinical research centre in Bethesda required that panels of scientists be formed to review the protocol of studies involving healthy volunteers. Other institutions were also beginning to convene informal groups of scientists to review the ethical aspects of research, but initially these did not include representatives from the community.

In 1962, as a result of the discovery that many of the women who had been prescribed thalidomide during pregnancy had not been told by their doctors that it was an experimental drug, amendments were made to the Food, Drug and Cosmetic Act to require that patients be informed of the experimental nature of new drugs and to give consent. Concern for the welfare of research subjects was heightened, in 1963, by the revelation that elderly patients at the Jewish Chronic Diseases Hospital in Brooklyn had been injected with cancer cells without being told.

Dr Henry K. Beecher, in 1966, raised ethical issues in an article in the *New England Journal of Medicine*. In a review of published research papers he identified instances of lack of appropriate treatment or questionable surgical procedures (Beecher 1966).

In 1972 attention was again focused on research subjects with the public disclosure of research on untreated syphilis in which 300 people in Alabama were denied treatment in order to investigate the natural course of the disease. As a result of Senate Hearings arising from this and other studies, Congress passed the Research Act of 1974. One of its requirements was the establishment of Institutional Review Boards to review all Department of Health and Welfare funded research. It also established the National Commission for the Protection of Human Subjects of Biomedical and Behavioral Research. The Commission issued a report in 1979, that summarises the basic ethical principles which underlie research. Drafted at a conference centre outside Baltimore – the Belmont Center – it became known as the Belmont Report (Belmont Report, 1979).

United Kingdom

In the UK in 1967, the Royal College of Physicians (RCP) recommended that all research on patients and healthy volunteers should be subject to ethical review. Its report was widely circulated by the Department of Health and many ethics committees were set up on an informal basis. The same year saw the publication of Pappworth's book, *Human Guinea Pigs, Experimentation on Man*, which highlighted concerns about the welfare of research subjects (Pappworth, 1967).

In 1973, the Chief Medical Officer of the Department of Health sought formal advice from the RCP on the composition and scope of research ethics committees. In 1975, the Department of Health endorsed the RCP's recommendations and advised health authorities on their implementation.

It was not until 1991, however, that the Department of Health formally required every health district to have a local medical research ethics committee and provided guidance on the composition of these committees and how they should function (Department of Health 1991).

General ethical principles

The three basic ethical principles, which should underlie all research on patients or healthy volunteers, were set out in the Belmont Report (1979). These principles, *respect for persons*, *beneficence* and *justice*, are widely accepted in society as a whole.

Respect for persons implies a respect for *autonomy*, or the right of people who are capable of making their own decisions to make those decisions for themselves. In accord with this principle, they should be provided with all the necessary information to help them make their decisions. In the ethics of research this means that patients and healthy volunteers should only enter studies after they have been provided with adequate information and freely given their informed consent.

Respect for persons also means protecting those who, because of extreme youth, mental disability or serious illness, are unable to make decisions for themselves. It may mean preventing them from doing things that might harm them or, in the research context, excluding them from certain kinds of study.

Beneficence refers to the ethical obligation to improve people's well-being and to do them no harm. The Hippocratic principle 'do no harm' has long been a fundamental principle of medical ethics. In terms of research, this principle underlines the importance of ensuring that the risks of the research are minimal in comparison with the potential benefits. Whether the potential benefits justify the risks is a central question facing those who must decide whether research projects can go ahead.

Justice refers to the obligation to treat everyone in accordance with what is 'right and proper', and to give each person what he or she is due. In research, this principle applies largely to ensuring that those who bear the discomforts and risks of research are the ones who stand to benefit. Thus it would be unacceptable to employ only disadvantaged subjects to test a new drug, which their poverty would deny them access to should it prove beneficial.

The philosophical principles underlying the ethics of medical research in particular and of medicine in general has been the subject of extensive debate. The reader interested in delving deeper into the subject is referred to the Further Reading list at the end of this book.

What is medical research?

Article I.2 of the Declaration of Helsinki emphasises the need for research protocols to be scrutinised by an independent medical research ethics committee. But what is research and how does it differ from standard clinical practice and medical audit?

Research versus standard clinical practice

A characteristic of *medical research* is that it is not necessarily intended to directly benefit the individuals taking part in it. Its aim is to: obtain more knowledge about the cause of disease and the working of the body in relation to disease; develop new treatments; or compare existing treatments with each other to see which is the more effective.

It may be known from the outset that at least some of the participants in the research will not themselves benefit. This will be the case when a drug trial includes a control group of patients receiving no active treatment and, even more obviously, in preliminary studies on a new drug involving healthy volunteers rather than patients. Basic research often does not involve direct medical care at all. It may, for example, simply involve taking blood or urine samples for analysis in an effort to obtain increased knowledge from which future patients may benefit.

Standard clinical practice, in contrast, involves using the treatment which the doctor thinks is most appropriate for the patients under his or her care, and is aimed at helping the individual patient. No patients – their general medical condition and resources allowing – will be left without treatment.

Research should be described in a formal protocol that states the aims of the study and describes the methods, whereas standard clinical practice is not usually so rigorously documented, although it is becoming increasingly so. The research protocol usually commits the researcher to a standard course of action which cannot be varied so readily as standard clinical care should the patient's condition undergo a significant change. When this occurs, the patient may have to be withdrawn from the study in order for alternative treatment to be implemented.

When the distinction becomes blurred

As standard clinical practice should be based on the evidence of well-designed and conducted research, it is obvious which should come first. Unfortunately, in the past, much that is now standard clinical practice was allowed to creep in without being adequately researched, leaving us uncertain just how effective some established treatments really are. As a result, the distinction between research and practice becomes blurred as research projects are designed to compare the effectiveness of different standard methods of treatment.

All of the patients in such studies will receive well-established treatments, which the doctor believes from experience will be of benefit to them, as would be the case in standard clinical practice. The scientifically designed comparison of the two treatments with the random allocation of patients to them, however, defines the activity as research. All such studies must be reviewed by an ethics committee.

Are all new procedures research?

The fact that a treatment is new, or different, or has not been properly tested before does not automatically make it research. It only becomes research if, in the words of the Declaration of Helsinki, it is, 'formulated in an experimental protocol', and compared in a formal way with other treatments or with no treatment, or a careful assessment is made of its safety and value to patients. Every new treatment or experimental procedure should become the object of formal research at an early stage in its development in order to ensure that it is safe and effective. Health authorities, hospitals and heads of department all have a responsibility to ensure that major innovations introduced by doctors in their area of influence are incorporated into formal research projects at the earliest possible opportunity.

Medical audit

A third kind of activity that is neither standard clinical practice nor research is known as medical audit. This activity is primarily concerned with assessing the quality of the care provided to patients in order to identify opportunities for improvement and to develop ways of bringing it about. Its activities range from considering the comfort of patients waiting for an outpatient appointment to identifying the cause of post-operative deaths. The audit may be carried out by the consultant and his team responsible for the care of the patients, or by someone from outside the hospital. Medical audit is seen as part of standard good practice in caring for patients and, except when it has the features described under 'If in doubt' below, does not require approval by a medical research ethics committee.

Unlike research, medical audit never involves the random allocation of patients to different treatment groups. Audit may well involve a comparison of different treatments, but the choice of treatment will have been made positively by the patients themselves after full discussion (ideally) of the known advantages and disadvantages, or by the doctor with the interests of individual patients in mind. The random allocation of patients to different treatment groups clearly defines an activity as research rather than medical audit.

Another useful distinction between research and audit is that while therapeutic research usually involves extra disturbance or work for the patients beyond that required for standard clinical care, medical audit rarely does so. The most that is usually involved is an interview or non-intrusive questionnaire asking for their views on the treatment that they have received.

Subtle distinctions
The distinction between standard clinical care, medical audit and research can be subtle. Suppose for example that a researcher wanted an answer to the question: 'what proportion of patients with stroke or peripheral vascular disease also have undiagnosed heart problems?' In a hospital where the appropriate diagnostic heart scan is performed routinely on all patients presenting with any kind of cardiovascular or cerebrovascular disease, it should be possible to answer the question from standard clinical case notes. This is little more than medical audit although a research type question is being asked and so long as strict standards of confiden-

tiality are adhered to, it is unlikely that it will raise any serious ethical issues. If, however, the hospital does not perform these tests routinely and they are done specifically to answer the question, this would fall clearly within the definition of research and need to be reviewed by a medical research ethics committee.

If in doubt

Definitions fail to cover every eventuality and if the investigator is in any doubt about whether an activity constitutes research or not, the rule is that he or she should, as required by Article I.2 of the Declaration of Helsinki, submit it for review by an independent ethics committee.

While medical audit will often not require scrutiny by an ethics committee, it will do so when potential breaches of confidentiality, intrusive questions or extra tests are involved. It may mean visiting patients in their home and administering questionnaires. This could raise additional ethical issues including the possibility of raising false expectations or re-awakening awareness of their illness.

There would also seem to be little logic in excluding experimental procedures from ethical review simply because they have not been incorporated into a formal research project and some ethics committees have broadened their remit to include these. If there is the slightest doubt, the appropriate ethics committee should be approached for advice as early as possible during the design of the study.

2

Medical research ethics committees: protecting patients, researchers and institutions

Article I.2 of the Declaration of Helsinki (World Medical Association 1996) states:

> The design and performance of each experimental procedure involving human subjects should be clearly formulated in an experimental protocol which should be transmitted for consideration, comment and guidance to a specially appointed committee independent of the investigator and the sponsor.

Who decides what research can be done on patients?

As we have already observed, it was traditionally left to doctors themselves to decide what research was acceptable to do on their patients or healthy volunteers and whether the risks justified the potential benefits. When the doctors who wish to conduct research into a particular condition are recognised experts in its treatment, are they not indeed the best people to decide what is acceptable for their patients? While this may well be the case, there is still a need to ensure that over enthusiastic researchers do not get so carried away with making a valuable contribution to science, and improving the lot of patients in the future, that they fail to ensure adequately the safety and comfort of patients today.

Local research ethics committees and their role

Before it can get underway, new research involving patients or healthy volunteers has, in accord with Article I.2 of the Declaration of Helsinki, to be clearly formulated in an experimental protocol and approved by a committee independent of the investigator and the sponsor. In the UK these committees are known as local research ethics committees, while in the USA, the institutional review boards serve this function. In the UK, a system of multicentre research ethics committees has recently been set up to review multicentre studies being conducted at sites in five or more local research ethics committee areas. For the purposes of this publication, these committees will collectively be referred to as ethics committees.

It should be emphasised at the outset, that our discussion is confined to *research* ethics committees, not those committees that decide who is going into the dialysis programme, who is a potential transplant recipient and so on, which though rare in the UK, are more common in the USA.

Duties of an ethics committee

The ethics committee has an important moral and social responsibility. Scientific research is permitted by Western society to advance medical knowledge but concern for the safety of the patient/volunteer must never be lost in a consideration of the potential benefits to be gained.

The first duty of an ethics committee is to protect the interests of patients, secondly to protect researchers and thirdly to protect the good name of the institution in which the research is being carried out (Royal College of Physicians 1996, s.1.5–1.7):

► Patients must be protected from undue risk of injury, distress or discomfort. They have a right to know what is being done to them and why, and their freedom of choice, confidentiality and privacy must be respected. Research participants should have direct access to the research ethics committee if they are dissatisfied (Royal College of Physicians 1996, s.5.24).

► Researchers must be protected from litigation or adverse publicity, or damage to their careers, by ensuring that at all times their research is carried out with due regard to professional regulations and guidelines, that informed consent is always obtained when feasible and that ethics approval is obtained prior to initiating or modifying the research.

► The reputation of the institution similarly stands to suffer if its employees do not meet these requirements.

Who should be responsible for setting up ethics committees?

The World Health Organization (WHO) guidelines state that: 'review committees may be created under the aegis of national or local health administrations, national medical research councils or other nationally-representative bodies' (CIOMS/WHO 1993, g.14).

The UK government decided (Department of Health 1991, s.2.1) that responsibility for the setting up of ethics committees should lie with the local health authorities, known in England and Wales as district health authorities, in Scotland as health boards and in Northern Ireland as health and social services boards. Most local research ethics committees, like the health authorities, therefore cover several hospitals and other research institutions and general practices. This arrangement broadly satisfies the UK requirement for ethics committees to be independent of the research institutions or hospitals where the research is being carried out. In the USA, there is no such requirement for the physical separation of the ethics committee from the institution in which the research is conducted, although institutional review board decisions must not of course be influenced by factors such as the desire of the institution to obtain research funding.

Some multinational companies, as for example Unilever, have their own network of ethics committees (Anon, 1996a). In Unilever these are under the guidance of a central ethical compliance group, set up to maintain uniformly high standards and best practices amongst the ethics committees, review and disseminate its own guidelines and provide ethical advice to committees and the company board. This has the advantage of ensuring ethical review of projects in parts of the world where the local system may be inadequate.

The investigator must obtain formal ethical approval *before* the research is begun (CIOMS/WHO 1993, g.14). It is important not to enter patients in a study in anticipation of approval.

The local medical research ethics committee will review the research proposal at one of its regular meetings, which should be held at frequent intervals. In the UK, it is recommended that meetings should be held each calendar month (Bendall 1994, p.16.) A number of responses to a proposal are possible. If it is considered acceptable, the committee may formally approve it, or approve it conditional on minor amendments being made. If not, they may defer it to a future meeting of the committee to obtain further information from the researchers or an outside expert. If the proposal is clearly unsatisfactory in its present form, they may ask for it to be revised and resubmitted, or reject it outright. Where an adverse decision is recorded it should be accompanied by an explanation of the reasons for rejection and advice to the applicant, who should be able to submit a revised proposal (45 CFR, 46.109d). If the applicant and committee feel it would be helpful, researchers should be given the opportunity to appear before the committee to explain the study in detail and respond to questions. The discussion should always be carried out in a way that is helpful and educative. The committee should produce its response with the minimum of delay.

A typical local medical research ethics committee constitution and mode of operation can be found in Appendix 2.

Who should sit on an ethics committee?

Who sits on an ethics committee and how qualified are they to assess the value of research proposals and their impact on patients? There is no consensus on exactly how many members should make up an ethics committee, only that they should collectively have the qualifications and experience to review and evaluate the science, medical aspects and ethics of the proposed trial. The International Conference on Harmonisation (ICH) good clinical practice guidelines (ICH 1996) and the US Department of Health and Human Services (DHHS) regulations (45 CFR, 46.107a; 21 CFR, 56.107a) state a minimum of five. In view of the difficulty of achieving the wide range of skills and experience required in five members, even if they are all present at a meeting, the Department of Health guidelines, which state that ethics committees in England and Wales should have between 8 and 12 members would seem more realistic (Department of Health 1991, s.2.4). There is universal agreement, however, that members should be drawn from both sexes (CIOMS/WHO 1993, g.14; Royal College of Physicians 1996, s.4.6; 45 CFR, 46.107b; 21 CFR 56.107b).

Ideally, ethics committees should include representatives of the major specialities practised within the area so that there is at least one expert capable of assessing the scientific value of the study and the safety of the class of drugs or of the techniques to which the participants will be exposed. The large number of specialities makes this difficult to achieve in practice, as specialisation in medicine is such that, for instance, an orthopaedic surgeon may know very little about obstetrics and gynaecology or vice versa.

As many studies come from general medical practice in countries where the family doctor system operates, or involve patients being exposed to treatments of which their family doctor should be aware, one committee member should also be a family doctor, preferably active, but if this is not possible, recently retired. Similarly, a nurse who is in day-to-day contact with patients in the community or on the wards and primarily concerned with their welfare is an essential component of any committee. For basic research of a highly technical nature, an experienced researcher other than a doctor, with a knowledge of biochemistry or pharmacology and statistics who can assess whether the design of the research proposal is adequate for it to yield any useful information, is also a valuable asset to a committee, particularly if employed as a scientific adviser.

The importance of lay members

The importance of lay members is universally recognised (Department of Health 1991, s.2.5; CIOMS/WHO 1993, g.14; ICH 1996, s.3.2.1; Royal College of Physicians 1996, s.4.6). The ICH and American regulations state that committees should have at least one member whose primary area of interest is non-scientific and that at least one member should have no connection with the institution concerned (ICH 1996 s.3.2.1.; 45 CFR, 46.107c–d; 21 CFR, 56.107c–d), but do not specify that they should be different people. Ethics committees in the UK are required to include at least two lay members, at least one of whom should have no connection at all with the health service (Department of Health 1991, s.2.7; Royal College of Physicians 1996, s.4.6). The average lay membership of UK ethics committees is currently three, out of an average membership of 11 to 12 (Nicholson 1997a). Without lay members, the committee may be open to the criticism – probably unfair, as doctors are the fiercest critics of other doctors – that it is an 'old boy's network' of researchers assessing each other's work.

The choice of lay members is always difficult. Ideally they should represent the public at large. In practice they are usually professional people, mainly because to handle the huge amount of paper work involved, perhaps 25 lengthy proposals a month, implies the sort of professional training in bulk paper handling that a doctor or lawyer receives. The second problem arises from the fact that ethics committee membership, at least in the UK, is generally regarded as a public service, and as such receives no financial remuneration (although this may be changing). It would usually be more difficult for say a brick layer to get paid time off work to sit on an ethics committee than for a university professor who has more control over his working week and can justify participation as an extension of his academic activities. This is a pity because people with less formal academic training are just as likely as the professional to make sound ethical decisions, relying more perhaps on gut feelings, rather than being unduly swayed by knowledge of published guidelines or current practice. On the other hand, the Royal College of Physicians makes the point that lay members should 'be persons of responsibility and standing who will not be overawed by medical members' (Royal College of Physicians 1996, s. 4.3).

A problem facing lay members of an ethics committee is the jargon-filled language that biomedical scientists and doctors, in common with most professionals, typically use to describe their work. Although the committee may require researchers to provide a one-page summary of their proposed research in their own words in language suitable for both medical and lay members of the committee, many researchers have great difficulty writing plain, jargon-free English (for help, see Goodman and Edwards 1997). The employment of a scientific or medical advisor, who may also be a committee member, to help lay members interpret the scientific basis and language of studies has been found to be of considerable help in this respect.

Is one committee enough?

The workload of ethics committees in the UK continues to rise. Over four times as many projects were reviewed in 1995 as in 1982, with the number of proposals considered per committee reaching an average of around 120 per year (Nicholson 1997a). In areas with a very strong research base, more than one committee may be required to handle the workload. This provides the opportunity for the creation of specialised sub-committees. In Scotland, the Lothian Research Ethics Committee, which deals with over 400 applications each year, has taken this course of action and created the following subcommittees, the activities of which are overseen by the main committee: medicine; surgery; anaesthetics/dentistry;

paediatric/reproductive medicine; general practice/public health medicine; and psychiatry/ psychology.

Each subcommittee has the same number of lay and overall members as a typical main committee, but has the advantage that its clinical members are specialists in the areas of research which come to their attention.

Individuals of sound judgement

Although they may be drawn from established groups, it must be emphasised that committee members are *not* representatives of those groups and must never regard themselves as such, or be regarded as such by employers or colleagues.

As emphasised by the UK Department of Health guidelines: 'they are appointed in their own right as individuals of sound judgement and relevant experience' (Department of Health 1991, s.2.6).

Whenever there is conflict between the interest of the patient, and that of the committee member's institution or department, as may well be the case with insurance arrangements, the interest of the patient must always come first. When a member has a 'vested' interest in a proposal, as when it is submitted by themselves or a close colleague, once they have (if necessary) been directly questioned about the proposal, they must leave the meeting until it has been discussed. To avoid embarrassment, they should not expect to hear the outcome until the secretary conveys the committee's decision in writing in the normal way.

A list of ethics committee members with their qualifications and affiliations should be publicly available. In the USA, the list must be submitted to the Office for Protection from Research Risks (45 CFR, 46.103b3).

Secretarial support

In order to function efficiently, in view of the huge amount of paper work and general correspondence involved, the committee needs to be supported by a secretariat including an experienced administrator/secretary and a typist/general clerical assistant. It should also include a scientific and/or medical advisor who may or may not be a committee member. This is especially important when the chairperson is a lay member. Unfortunately, at the time of writing, many ethics committees do not receive this basic level of support.

Pharmaceutical companies need to be informed of the constitution of the ethics committees which approve their proposals to ensure that the approval is valid and will be accepted by the regulatory authorities in all of the countries in which they wish to obtain a product licence. Minimum standards of composition have been set by the ICH, good clinical practice guidelines that came into effect in January 1997 (ICH 1996, s.3.2.1). The regulatory authorities, therefore, currently play a background role in ensuring that the constitution of ethics committees meets the required standards in countries lacking regulations or official guidelines on this matter. As their influence is largely restricted to drug development trials, there is a further requirement for government health departments to ensure, as does the Department of Health in England and Wales, the Scottish Office in Scotland, the Northern Ireland Office in Northern Ireland and the DHHS in the USA, that the composition of committees meets the required standards.

How long should committee members serve?

The Department of Health guidelines state that committee members should be appointed to serve for a period of three to five years (Department of Health 1991 s.2.9). Though not mentioned in the guidelines, there may be a case for probationary appointments of three to six months during which the appointee and the committee consider whether they are able to commit the time and are contributing effectively. Otherwise committees are faced with an empty chair, nothing to say, or 'sorry, but I'm on call' problem. In considering whether to renew an effective individual's membership for another period, the possibility that a member may become unduly influential has to be balanced against the advantages of having experienced, committed members on the committee.

The chairperson and vice-chairperson

The Department of Health guidelines (1991, s.2.8) state that either the chairperson or vice-chairperson, or possibly both, should be lay members of the ethics committee, a view supported by the Royal College of Physicians (1996, s.4.10). Whether medical or lay, the chairperson needs to exercise considerable skill to counteract the natural tendency for meetings to be dominated by the expert members and to ensure that lay members are encouraged to express their views. The development of true consensus views without having any particular individual, medical or lay, dominating proceedings is essential. Most lay chairpersons will need professional advice to assist them in taking chairperson's action, and if the vice-chairperson is not medically qualified a scientific and/or medical advisor will need to be appointed to assist the chairperson. There is no obvious ethical reason why advisors should not be committee members, but some health organisations have rules that do not allow advisors of their various committees to also serve as members.

In the UK, health authorities have typically appointed the chairperson and vice-chairperson of local research ethics committees, (like those of most health service committees) directly from the community, sometimes following a public advertisement. In view of the increasing complexity of the ethical issues that have to be dealt with, it is becoming increasingly difficult to appoint external candidates with the necessary experience. It may now be more appropriate, where feasible, for the local health authority, or committee itself, to appoint their own chairpersons from amongst their membership, as is indeed recommended by the Department of Health (1991, s.2.8).

What constitutes a quorum?

At least half of the members should be present, at least one of whom should be lay and two medically qualified (Bendall 1994, p.15; 45 CFR, 46.108b; 21 CFR, 56.108c).

Evaluation of a research proposal

What aspects of a proposal does an ethics committee assess?

Firstly, the protocol must be scientifically sound and properly designed so that the information being sought can in fact be obtained by the methods to be used. The WHO guidelines state that 'normally ethical review committees consider both the scientific and ethical aspects of proposed research' (CIOMS/WHO 1993, g.14), and the institutional review boards and research ethics committees have traditionally performed this task.

The Royal College of Physicians guidelines (1996, s. 2.1–2.3), while taking the view that the main role of an ethics committee should be to scrutinise projects from an ethical standpoint, recognises that they are often placed in the unsatisfactory position of having to assess their scientific validity as well. While a study that is so badly designed as to be incapable of yielding any worthwhile results is, by definition, unethical it is questionable whether prime responsibility for assessing the scientific validity of a study should be imposed on the local ethics committee. Although committees will naturally feel a responsibility for assessing the scientific merit of a study, they cannot be expected to have within their ranks a sufficient range of expertise in all branches of medical science to be able to assess in all cases whether it is potentially capable of making a contribution to knowledge. In some cases, it may be obvious to scientific members that the design of a study is flawed but other studies may require expert assessment. When studies initiated by doctors and hospital researchers are submitted to major national grant awarding bodies for funding, as for example in Britain, the Medical Research Council, assessment of scientific validity will be made by experts before the study goes ahead.

Where studies are to be financed out of an institution's own financial allocations, or small private and charitable funds, rather than by a major funding body with its network of expert referees, there is a need for an effective mechanism for ensuring adequate peer review before a proposal comes before an ethics committee. One such mechanism is currently under development in Teaching Hospital National Health Service Trusts in Britain motivated by the government's desire that funds allocated by them for research and development should be more rigorously accounted for. The intention is that all research on human subjects involving health service staff, premises or other major facilities will be screened for its scientific validity by a specially formed research and development office before being passed onto the ethics committee for ethical review.

The ethics committee should determine whether an assessment of scientific validity of the study has already been made, or whether it will be a prerequisite of funding. Where a rigorous system of peer review is currently lacking, ethics committees are often taking on a bigger role in assessing the scientific validity of studies than they should have to. The committees need to emphasise to institutions the importance of developing such a system for studies being conducted on their premises or by their employees.

The ICH good clinical practice guidelines (ICH 1996 s.3) includes a list of those aspects of a trial apart from its scientific validity that should be evaluated by the ethics committee.

Standard proposal form

To obtain consistent answers to key questions so that studies can be effectively evaluated, ethics committees need to have a standard form on which proposals for research are submitted to them.

As yet in the UK, there is no standard proposal form for use by all local committees – each having its own cherished version. This has long been a source of irritation to researchers involved in multicentre studies and was a major factor behind the drive for the introduction of multicentre research ethics committees with a nationally accepted standard form. In practice many local committees are willing to accept another committee's form when it is clearly impracticable for researchers to complete a separate form for every committee to which they must apply, as with epidemiologists studying rare diseases who have to cast their net nationwide.

What the committee needs to know

The specimen ethics committee proposal form reproduced in Appendix 3 is designed to elicit the required information. What is required and why is summarised briefly below, with each aspect being considered in greater detail in later chapters.

Details of the researchers

Both international (Commission of the European Communities 1990 s.1.6a; CIOMS/WHO 1993, g.14; ICH 1996, s.3.1.3) and national (Royal College of Physicians 1996, s.2.6) guidelines emphasise the importance of ensuring that the researcher is qualified to carry out the proposed research. The local research ethics committee will wish to satisfy itself on the following points.

► The investigator must have appropriate professional qualifications and research experience and be fully familiar with the techniques of the research and, in drug trials, with the properties of the medicine being used.

► In order to decide whether the investigator has sufficient time to conduct and complete the study, the committee will need to know how may other studies he or she is currently involved in.

► Any associated researchers must be clearly identified, and the committee kept informed of changes.

In order to assess whether the facilities are adequate, the committee will need details of the premises in which the study will be undertaken.

The local research ethics committee will also need to know who is the senior clinician responsible for the study. As the responsibility of a doctor for his patients includes the research he allows to be carried out on them, the name and address of the doctor responsible for the care of the patients, if different from the researcher, should also be provided.

With the recent creation of a network of multicentre research ethics committees in the UK, the role of *local* research ethics committees in assessing local matters such as the adequacy of facilities has been given greater emphasis (Department of Health 1997a, b).

Sponsor/source of funding/financial matters

The committee will need to know who is sponsoring the project. If charges are to be made to commercial companies for the ethical review of their studies, the committee will need details to supply to the finance department of the organisation that will be receiving the payment.

Questions regarding financial arrangements arise out of the need to ensure that researchers are not put under any undue pressure to recruit patients to the study or to retain them once recruited. Financial arrangements between an investigator and the sponsor should allow pro rata payments for the work done and not depend on patients completing the trial or a predetermined number of patients having to be recruited. Fees should not exceed the hourly rates recommended by the appropriate professional bodies. The committee will need to know into what fund the money will be credited and the purpose for which the fund will be used.

The committee will also need to know the amount being paid to volunteers to ensure that it does not constitute an inducement to participate against their better judgement. At the same time, they will need to be reassured that patients or volunteers are being fairly recompensed for out-of-pocket expenses incurred as a result of their participation.

Classification of the research

From information that is given about the type of participant – for example healthy volunteer or inpatient – type of research and general purpose of the study, the committee can form a broad picture of the pattern of research in its area and how it varies over time.

Previous assessment

Committees should not work in isolation. It is of interest to a committee to know whether a proposal turned down by itself has been approved by another committee or conversely whether another committee has turned down a proposal which it sees no good reason to refuse and to try to establish the reasons for the discrepancy.

Details of the research

The researcher is asked to provide details of the research, including a one-page A4 (i.e. 210 × 297 mm or 8.27 × 11.69 in.) summary of the background and justification for the research and what it will actually involve for participants, in language comprehensible to both medical and lay members.

Participants

This section of the proposal form is designed to provide the committee with information regarding the number and age range of participants. The very young and very old will arouse particular concerns as will the possibility that subjects are in a dependent relationship with the researcher, which might lead to undue pressure to participate.

Obtaining informed consent

Informed consent is the central ethical issue in research. In view of the overriding importance of obtaining, in all but the most exceptional of cases, the informed consent of participants, the committee will need the following information to enable it to assess whether or not the consent procedure is adequate. Will the committee's standard consent form be used? Who will provide the information and seek consent from the patient/carer? How and when will subjects first be approached with information about the study? How much time will be allowed for discussion with relatives, friends or the family doctor before giving consent? Are any patients likely to have problems in giving informed consent because of age, intellectual disability, mental illness or severity of illness? If so, how will the consent process be managed?

Influence of the research on the normal treatment of patients

In order to ensure that the patients' treatment is not being adversely affected by their participation in a trial, the committee will seek through its proposal form to obtain answers to the following questions. If prospective participants are on long-term medication for their condition and it is to be discontinued, what is the ethical justification for this? What percentage of participants will be on placebo medication and for how long? What rescue medication will be available? What are the plans for treating patients at the end of the formal trial? Are patients themselves likely to benefit from participation in the study?

Hazards and discomforts

In order to assist the committee in its assessment of risks and hazards, this section asks for the nature of any additional invasive procedures to be used in the study. It asks for details of the potential risks associated with them, or with the withholding of treatment. It also asks what discomforts may be experienced, and what steps are taken to minimise them.

Medicines involved

In the case of studies involving the administration of drugs, details of strengths and dose frequency and route of administration are requested, with a summary of known toxic effects on humans. The proposal form also asks whether the research involves radioactive materials or X-rays or the administration of a new, non-formulary drug, and if so, for confirmation that the appropriate certificates have been, or will be, obtained from the regulatory authorities.

Confidentiality

Breaches of confidentiality can have serious consequences for participants, affecting their relationships, social status or their job. What steps, therefore, are being taken to ensure the confidentiality of patients and volunteers?

Indemnity arrangements

The ethics committee will wish to ensure that participants are adequately insured should anything go wrong in the study. Researchers are asked to state the nature of their insurance and indemnity arrangements and whether participants will be covered by 'no fault' insurance.

Who should complete the proposal form?

The researcher in charge of the project should complete the proposal form. A researcher who has not prepared a research proposal for an ethics committee before, should seek the assistance of an experienced colleague both in completing the form and in designing an effective patient or volunteer information sheet. Each department or institution should designate an experienced researcher to offer guidance to new recruits in preparing proposals. So often, new researchers are left to their own devices with a consequent needless waste of time and effort for all concerned when proposals are initially rejected for failing to provide the basic information on which the committee can base an assessment.

The senior clinician with overall responsibility for the project should always carefully scrutinise the proposal form before countersigning it to ensure that it has been satisfactorily completed.

Although it simplifies matters for local investigators, it is not really satisfactory for ethics committee proposal forms to be completed in their entirety by drug company representatives, as the description of the project provided by local investigators gives the ethics committee some indication of their understanding of it. With the introduction of multicentre ethics committees, however, ensuring individual researcher input into proposals for drug development studies becomes increasingly difficult.

In addition to the proposal form, researchers must submit copies of the information sheet and the consent form they intend to give to participants, letters to family doctors and any questionnaires or advertisements that will be used. Where applicable, certificates from medicines control agencies, radiation protection committees, etc. and, in the case of drug trials, pharmaceutical company protocols and investigator brochures should also be submitted.

Chairperson's action/expedited review

New proposals

Should all proposals for research be put before the whole ethics committee or can some types of research be decided by chairperson's action/expedited review?

It must be emphasised that expedited review is not the same thing as bland acceptance of certain kinds of study. The proposal form must be completed with the same thoroughness as if it were going to the whole committee and the methods of obtaining consent must be no less satisfactory. The only difference is that it is the chairperson with advice, if necessary, from individual members, or a member designated by the chairperson, rather than the whole committee, who, after careful consideration of the proposal, gives the initial decision for it to go ahead (45 CFR, 46.110 and 21 CFR, 56.110). If they feel they cannot approve it themselves, it must then go to the whole committee.

In the UK, the Royal College of Physicians (1996, s.5.10) is cautious about the potential for chairperson's action, suggesting only that 'investigations which pose no ethical problems and are without risk of distress or injury, psychological or physical, to the subjects, e.g. some epidemiology, some surveys of the public's eating habits, assessment of patient information and education' may qualify. It emphasises that wherever there is any doubt, the application should go to the full committee.

This contrasts with the much bolder attitude to expedited review on the other side of the Atlantic. In February 1997, the Office for Protection from Research Risks in the USA reissued the following statement in regard to expedited review.

> Research activities involving no more than **minimal** risk *and* in which the only involvement of human subjects will be in one or more of the following categories (carried out through standard methods) may be reviewed by the Institutional Review Board through the expedited review procedure.
>
> 1 Collection of hair and nail clippings, in a non-disfiguring manner; deciduous teeth, and permanent teeth if patient care indicates a need for extraction.
> 2 Collection of excreta and external secretions including sweat, uncannulated saliva, placenta removed at delivery, and amniotic fluid at the time of rupture of the membrane prior to or during labor.
> 3 Recording of data from subjects 18 years of age and older using non-invasive procedures routinely employed in clinical practice. This includes the use of physical sensors that are applied either to the surface of the body or at a distance and do not involve input of matter or significant amounts of energy into the subject or an invasion of the subject's privacy. It also includes such procedures as

weighing, testing sensory acuity, electrocardiography, electroencephalography, thermography, detection of naturally occurring radioactivity, diagnostic echography, and electroretinography. It does not include exposure to electromagnetic radiation outside the visible range (for example, X-rays, microwaves).

4 Collection of blood samples by venepuncture, in amounts not exceeding 450 millilitres in an eight week period and no more often than two times per week, from subjects 18 years of age or older and who are in good health and not pregnant.

5 Collection of both supra- and subgingival dental plaque and calculus, provided the procedure is not more invasive than routine prophylactic scaling of the teeth and the process is accomplished in accordance with accepted prophylactic techniques.

6 Voice recordings made for research purposes such as investigations of speech defects.

7 Moderate exercise by healthy volunteers.

8 The study of existing data, documents, records, pathological specimens, or diagnostic specimens.

9 Research on individual or group behavior or characteristics of individuals, such as studies of perception, cognition, game theory, or test development, where the investigator does not manipulate subjects' behavior and the research will not involve stress to subjects.

10 Research on drugs or devices for which an investigational new drug exemption or an investigational device exemption is not required.

The trouble with expedited review

Many of the above categories of research, while appearing to carry no risk of injury, may pose wider ethical issues in regard to confidentiality and the religious and spiritual beliefs of patients. As these aspects will be discussed at length in later chapters, suffice it to mention here that hair clippings can be used to estimate past drug misuse, spare blood samples for testing for inherited defects with profound implications for patients and their relatives, and a placenta for developing agents of abortion. Seemingly innocuous studies may therefore carry profound ethical implications, which in my view will usually need to be discussed more fully by the whole committee and not left to the judgement of an individual. It may also be considered unfair to impose the additional burden of expedited review on the chairperson, particularly if he or she is part-time and unremunerated.

As chairperson's action will always have to be ratified by the full committee at its next meeting there remains the possibility that the chairperson's decision may be overturned. When there is any possibility of disagreement with the chairperson's decision, expedited review should be discouraged. The alternative is for chairperson's action to be absolute with the committee having to go along with the decision regardless of the consensus opinion. This would not generally be considered an option.

Chairperson's action is wholly appropriate when the full committee has required minor changes to a proposal and the researcher responds in writing agreeing to and showing evidence of the changes. The proposal may then be approved by the chairperson without needing to go back to the full committee. Indeed, when the changes requested by the committee are very minor, such as the inclusion in the patient information sheet of standard wording regarding the right to withdraw, the revised sheet may be approved by the committee secretary without needing to go to the chairperson. While a chairperson may give approval, a proposal can only be rejected following consideration by the full committee (45 CFR, 46.110b2).

Charging for submissions to local research ethics committees

At the time of writing, about a half of ethics committees in the UK make a charge, typically of around £250 for the ethical review of studies sponsored by commercial companies, and the number who do so is increasing rapidly.

The professional bodies and government departments in the UK have generally had little to say on this issue. The Royal College of Physicians (1996, s.5.25) states simply, 'In the case of direct applications from the private medical sector or other non-NHS source, a handling charge should be made, but it should cover no more than the relevant administration costs of the research ethics committee and is often waived for universities, charities and similar institutions'. Some thoughts on the subject are considered further.

Is it ethical for research ethics committees to charge for submissions?

It can be argued that charging is unethical in that it introduces a contract between the ethics committee and the researchers. If charging is considered, it should be done within the closely defined limits outlined below. The most important requirement is that it should in no way restrict or inhibit those who wish to initiate ethical medical research. Neither should a charge be so high as to influence a pharmaceutical company in its choice of locations for multicentre research.

Charging may have one or both of the following objectives:

▶ To help cover the significant costs involved in servicing an ethics committee. Funding is required for providing adequate administrative and clerical backup and for training members. It may also be needed to compensate departments and medical practices for the work lost while members are involved in the work of the ethics committee, and for providing remuneration, or at least out-of-pocket expenses, for retired or unemployed members.

▶ To discourage abuse of committee members' time by discouraging incompetent and inadequate submissions and those made speculatively without consideration of whether suitable patients for recruitment are available.

To achieve the second objective could mean penalising the majority of low budget studies in order to weed out a small minority of grossly inadequate submissions.

To avoid inhibiting research, the following submissions should *not* be subject to a charge:

- ▶ Medical research initiated by non-commercial investigators for the purpose of furthering scientific knowledge, whether paid for from departmental funds, by governmental or charitable grant-giving bodies, or other similar sponsors.
- ▶ Multicentre clinical trials or surveys under the auspices of non-commercial organisations, such as the Medical Research Council, or cancer charities.

The following may be subject to a charge:

- ▶ Multicentre clinical trials whose purpose is to provide data for a commercial sponsor for the purpose of drug or product development.
- ▶ Singlecentre trials of new drugs or products where the investigator is under contract and is receiving payment, or goods and services.

There should be a standard charge for the first submission, plus an additional charge if the committee considers that the initial documentation was substantially unsatisfactory so that it has to be reconsidered. A further charge could be levied for any subsequent significant protocol amendments needing to be considered by the committee, but many committees will not consider this worth the administrative hassle.

The fee will be for submission of a proposal and it will not be refundable if the research does not proceed.

The principal criteria for determining whether a submission fee is appropriate will be whether:

- ▶ the investigator is receiving a fee or significant payment in goods or services for the trial.

▶ the data are being generated for the benefit of a large commercial sponsor, rather than primarily for the interest of the local investigator.

(Research sponsored by very small companies, for example one set up by a nurse to develop a new aid for the disabled for which a need has been identified, may be excluded from charging.)

The decision as to whether or not a specific proposal attracts a submission fee will be obvious in most cases. Where there is potential hardship, or controversy, no committee should allow the existence of the fee to delay or inhibit potentially valuable research. An ethics committee should not delay consideration of a proposal pending receipt of the fee. Neither should approval be withheld if the fee is not paid.

Collecting the fee

The secretary of the committee, on advice from the chairperson, should indicate to the finance department of the health authority those companies to be invoiced. Responsibility for collection of the fee then passes entirely to the finance department. No one should expect the committee to bring any pressure to bear on defaulters. In my view, debt collection is not an appropriate activity for an ethics committee.

Ensuring value for money

If pharmaceutical companies and other sponsors are required to pay a significant fee for ethical review of their proposals, they have a right to expect an efficient service. It is prudent that income from charging is seen to be used to enhance the efficient functioning of the committee and not simply go into the general coffers of the organisation funding the committee's administration. At the same time it would surely be unethical to give any form of priority – for example, enhanced speed of response following the meeting, to those researchers or companies that are asked to pay, over those who are not.

Potential weak points in the system of local research ethics committees

Lack of consistency?

Would different committees presented with the same research proposal, express the same concerns, require the same amendments and come to the same final decision, or would it be accepted by some and rejected by others? In view of our familiarity with the wide range of sentences imposed by different law courts for essentially the same crime, total consistency amongst ethics committees is an unrealistic expectation. Complaints regarding the inconsistencies of ethics committees have been published in professional journals on a number of occasions by the organisers of multicentre trials.

A typical example of this is a postal survey aimed at comparing the health of children of different birth weights. This proposal was submitted to 162 local research ethics committees in England and Wales. Of these, 17 committees said it was not necessary to approach them for approval and 82 formally approved the study without comment. Others, however, raised a number of issues, including concerns about the study's aims, its costs, confidentiality, consent and the wording of questionnaires and information sheets, while 31 asked for the proposal to be revised and resubmitted (Middle et al. 1995).

Consistency is undoubtedly a problem and patients have no way of knowing how well their interests are being served by the committee operating in their area. As with any organisation, some committees are likely to be more thorough, and offer a greater degree of protection than others. The degree of protection afforded by a local ethics committee will depend on its structure, its expertise in the kind of study being proposed, how much time individual members have available to study the proposals, and their training as well as the soundness of their ethical judgement.

The development of national training schemes for ethics committee members and frequent opportunities for committees to meet and share their experiences is essential if a degree of consistency is to be achieved. A robust system of auditing the performance of the ethics committees would also help to maintain standards and confidence in their performance.

Some experimentation may slip through the net

A major weakness of the current system as it operates in the UK, is that doctors are only obliged to submit for ethical review formal research projects. Any doctor is free to perform a new operation on a patient, or continue with an outmoded treatment when a more effective one is available, without reference to an ethics committee. Ironically, those doctors who are prepared to admit that they are not sure which treatment is best for their patients and who therefore design a trial to find out, are the ones who have to gain the approval of the ethics committee before they can proceed.

In at least two new areas of medicine – gene therapy, and animal to human transplantation – a more rational situation is developing. It has been deemed that *all* experimentation in gene therapy is to be regarded as research and subject to the same rigid controls as other kinds of research. Consequently, all proposals for attempts at gene therapy in humans must in the UK first be submitted to a national gene therapy advisory committee and subsequently to the appropriate local research ethics committees (Gene Therapy Advisory Committee 1994).

A similar situation will apply regarding animal to human transplantation, with all experimentation considered as research and needing to be submitted initially to a national advisory committee (Nuffield Council on Bioethics 1996), although in the UK it is agreed that it is not currently acceptable to move to trials involving human beings (Advisory Group on the Ethics of Xenotransplantation, 1997).

Local health authorities and hospitals have a responsibility to ensure that all major innovations introduced by doctors in their area are incorporated into formal research projects as soon as possible, so that they can be reviewed by a local research ethics committee. The remit of committees needs to be widened to include experimentation that does not fall within the strict definition of research.

Approval should not imply moral acceptability

An ethics committee usually restricts its assessments of a research proposal to the ethics or morality of the research as it affects the physical or mental health of the participants, their carers or the public health. The committee as a whole is unlikely to concern itself with more spiritual matters, even though individual committee members, mirroring society as a whole, might consider certain kinds of experimentation morally wrong. A typical example would be research aimed at developing methods of prenatal screening for genetic disorders which might, if successful, result in the option of aborting affected fetuses. Although individual members might abstain from the discussion, most ethics committees in the UK would not consider it within their power to prevent morally debatable areas of research of this kind from taking place in the hospitals and research establishments for which they have responsibility. It could be argued that local research ethics committees *should* have this right and be prepared to exercise it, especially in parts of the world where the general population, because of their religious or spiritual beliefs, would find certain kinds of research unacceptable.

The patient and assessment of morality

Participant information sheets in the UK sometimes include a statement to the effect that: 'the local research ethics committee has scrutinised this study and raised no objections from the point of view of medical ethics'. This may be regarded as manipulative or coercive and may also mislead participants into thinking that the broader moral issues have been considered. Approval by an ethics committee is not tantamount to approval by the Church or other moral guardian. For these reasons such statements should be avoided.

In order for patients to give informed consent, researchers must always make clear the long-term aims and moral issues that may be raised by their research where these are known. Patients can then make their own moral judgements as to whether or not they wish to take part in a study that for them may involve no more than donating a few extra millilitres of blood, but which has profound moral implications.

It is essential for ethics committees in scrutinising research proposals to ensure that the broader moral issues have been properly addressed.

The absence of effective sanctions against researchers and sponsors when approval is not requested or the committee's conditions of approval are ignored

In the UK there is no legislation specifically relating to ethics committees and no legal obligation for researchers to submit proposals to them. In practice they do so because: National Health Service bodies require it under Department of Health guidance; it is an administrative requirement of most hospitals and other employing institutions; grant awarding bodies require evidence of ethical approval before releasing funds; most journals require it before publication; and drug licensing authorities require it. Many researchers also welcome the advice and reassurance that ethical review can offer.

Ethics committees in the UK, in common with institutional review boards in the USA (45 CFR, 46.113; 21 CFR, 56.113), have the authority to suspend or terminate approval of research that is not being conducted according to their requirements or has been associated with unexpected serious adverse events, but what if the researchers refuse to comply with this or other directions?

The lack of authority to impose sanctions is recognised as a problem for ethics committees worldwide (CIOMS/WHO, 1993, g.14). Local research ethics committees in the UK are typical in having no authority to take legal action against researchers who repeatedly violate the terms of an approval. However, as advised by the Department of Health, 'If it comes to the attention of a committee that research is being carried out which it has not been asked to consider or which it has considered but its recommendations have been ignored, then the local research ethics committee should bring the matter to the attention of its appointing authority, the relevant National Health Service body and to the appropriate professional body' (Department of Health 1991, s.3.22). US regulations similarly require all interested parties to be informed of serious or continuing noncompliance with institutional review board decisions (45 CFR, 46.103b5; 21 CFR, 56.108b). In practice, few researchers would wish to risk having their reputation harmed in this way by failing to observe basic ethical procedures.

If the ethics committee is unhappy with a trial, that for example is sponsored by a pharmaceutical company, because it considers that it has no scientific validity and is merely a marketing exercise, it can in the UK make a complaint to the Association of British Pharmaceutical Industries who will investigate and report on the matter.

Recent experience of on-site monitoring of projects following ethics committee approval (Smith et al., 1997) revealed that the vast majority of researchers were eager to conduct, and to be seen to be conducting, their research to the highest possible standards, and to co-operate fully with their local ethics committee. Lapses were generally due to misunderstandings, or momentary carelessness rather than deliberate attempts to undermine the system of ethical review. Researchers were keen to put things right as soon as possible and to take steps to avoid similar problems arising in the future.

Despite this, there is no room for complacency. There is a clear need for ethics committees to have in place an effective mechanism for dealing with serious offences if and when they arise and with repeat offenders. A case could be argued for the introduction of a Research Subject Protection Act to formalise the protection of research subjects in the sort of way that the UK Data Protection Act offers protection to data subjects. Failure to submit a proposal to an ethics committee would then be on a par with failure to register with the Data Protection Registrar a database containing personal information.

Ethical review of multicentre research

The original position

Some drug trials and epidemiological studies are designed to be conducted at a number of sites in different parts of a country or even internationally. In the absence of special arrangements for the ethical appraisal of multicentre research, the proposal has to be submitted by the investigators to the local research ethics committees serving each area in which the participants are located. This places a considerable burden on the organisers of multicentre research and can cause unacceptable delays to potentially valuable research.

Investigators are faced with having to spend a great deal of time and effort in submitting applications often, as in the UK, on many different 'standard' application forms, to numerous ethics committees up and down the country. Frustration frequently results from requests from different committees for different, often incompatible, amendments to protocols. The procedures used by each of the local research ethics committees also differ.

In the case of low budget epidemiological studies on rare conditions where patients have to be recruited from virtually every part of a country in order to obtain sufficient numbers for a scientifically valid study, the prospect of having to obtain ethical approval from almost every local research ethics committee in that country (e.g. over 200 in the UK) may abort projects even before they begin. Pharmaceutical companies, although less likely to be daunted by the prospect of having to apply to large numbers of local committees are nevertheless involved in a great deal of extra work, and possibly expensive delays, as a result.

From the point of view of local ethics committees it means that numerous local committees are involved in considering the same proposal. There would therefore be potential advantages to having a multicentre committee that can ensure that a scientific assessment of studies has been conducted and start screening out dubious borderline multicentre studies, which often appear to a local committee to be mere marketing exercises.

In the USA, the Department of Health and Human Services (45 CFR, 46.114) and the Food and Drug Administration (21 CFR, 56.114) regulations permit institutions involved in multi-institutional studies to use methods of joint or co-operative review. In the UK there has tended to be little co-operation of this kind between local research ethics committees.

Streamlining the system

In order to streamline arrangements for the review of multicentre research by ethics committees, it is generally agreed that an effective system of multicentre ethical review is essential. A streamlined system needs to be consistent with the following principles.

- ► It must be more efficient, whilst safeguarding the public and patients at least as effectively as the current one.
- ► It must command the confidence of patients, the research community and local research ethics committees.
- ► Local research ethics committees must retain the right to decide whether the research should go ahead locally.

▶ It must cover all multinational and multicentre research in the National Health Service, including clinical trials, records based, qualitative, and health service economic research, and surveys. It should also be able to advise on health related non-NHS research.

In the UK, a consultative group established to develop proposals for changes in the system, presented its recommendations to health authorities and local research ethics committees for their consideration in May 1996, and by April 1997, a system of multicentre ethical review was implemented in Scotland (Multicentre Research Ethics Committee Scotland 1997; Scottish Office 1997), and began to be extended to the rest of the UK later that year (Anon 1997c). It should be emphasised that multicentre research ethics committees in the UK are designed to work alongside the local research ethics committees and do not have administrative control over them.

Each of the 11 multicentre research ethics committees in the UK (one each in Scotland, Wales and Northern Ireland, and eight in England) serves an average population of just over five million. Each multicentre research protocol is considered by the multicentre committee in the region in which the principal researcher is based. As most multicentre proposals originate from the pharmaceutical industry, this can create an uneven workload where, as is the case in the UK, the headquarters of most companies tend to be located in one part of the country. The advice of the multicentre committee in relation to a research proposal is subsequently communicated to local ethics committees in every locality involved, not just those within the host region.

Once the multicentre committee has approved the proposal, local committees have the opportunity to accept or reject the protocol for local reasons. Current advice is that under the ICH guidelines (ICH 1996), chairman's action by local research ethics committees does not meet the proposed requirements for clinical trials that are designed to generate data for submitting to the regulatory authorities (Department of Health 1998). Each local research

Figure 2.1
Multi-centre research ethics committee flowchart

▼

Step 1 Principle Research Worker submits proposal to Multi-Centre Research Ethics Committee (MREC) for the Region in which he/she is based, on standard form.

▼

Step 2 Designated MREC considers the proposal

(At Step 2 the MREC may discuss the proposal with the principal researcher and/or seek advice from an appropriate external expert).

▼

Step 3 Designated MREC issues decision to Principal Researcher

(If a negative decision is given the principal researcher may revise the proposal and re-submit as at Step 1. The MREC response form will give detailed reasons for approval or refusal of the application).

▼

Step 4 Principal Researcher sends protocol, completed MREC Application Form, and MREC Response Form together with *Supplementary Form for Local Arrangements* to Local Research Workers.

▼

Step 5 Local Research Worker sends the endorsed, completed MREC Application Form, and MREC Response Form, together with the completed and signed *Supplementary Form for Local Arrangements* to the appropriate Local Research Ethics Committee (LREC).

▼

Step 6 An 'Executive Subcommittee' of the LREC considers issues affecting local acceptability.

(At Step 6, LRECs may discuss the proposal with the local and/or principal researcher and consider certain local issues. LRECs may also raise significant general concerns with the MREC through the administrator).

▼

Step 7 LREC advises local researchers, and the relevant MREC of its decision. LREC sends copy of its response and copy of the *Supplementary Form* to MREC, together with any comments.

(LRECs may approve or reject a proposal for strictly defined local reasons but not amend it apart from changes, where essential, to the patient information sheet to reflect local needs. In the event of rejection, detailed reasons should be given.).

▼

Step 8 The MREC considers local comments/decisions and may amend its decision in the light of these.

ethics committee is therefore required to establish a standing executive subcommittee, consisting of at least two members, specifically to consider multicentre research ethics committee proposals. On receipt of a multicentre research ethics committee approved application from a local researcher, a meeting of the local executive subcommittee must be called within two weeks. The meeting and the decision of the local executive subcommittee must be minuted and communicated in writing to the researcher within five working days, and a copy of the letter sent to the appropriate medical research ethics committee. They must give detailed reasons if they refuse a proposal.

What issues are the executive subcommittee asked to consider on behalf of the LREC?

According to the Department of Health advice, consideration should be limited to local issues including: (a) the experience of the researchers and their ability to carry out the number of studies in which they are involved; (b) the suitability of the local site and available facilities; (c) the suitability of the subjects, particularly in regard to the over-exploitation of specific groups of patients who are in high demand as research subjects.

In regard to the patient information sheet and consent form, the local research ethics committee executive subcommittee will need to check that local information, such as contact numbers and addresses, are appropriately inserted. They may advise on whether the information sheet and consent form need to be produced in languages other than English. No other changes may be requested to the information sheet or consent form, as doing so affects the integrity of the protocol. If it identifies strong ethical issues regarding a proposal, which it believes have not been adequately dealt with by the multicentre committee, the local executive subcommittee has a duty to draw its attention to them. If the multicentre committee realises that a serious oversight has occurred it may then suspend approval of the study at all sites. This should avoid the unacceptable situation which has on occasions occurred, where a multicentre study rejected by some local committees as unethical was allowed to proceed at other sites where the committees were less rigorous. A national database of proposals being set up by the multicentre committees will prevent sponsors who have had their project rejected by one multicentre committee from submitting it to other multicentre committees in the hope of finding one that will let it through. A European-wide database of clinical trials is also being established. The European Commission initially rejected the idea of a European-wide system of multicentre ethics committees, but may look at the possibility again.

The new system does not necessarily save pharmaceutical companies time, as they must now wait for central approval followed by local approval whereas previously some local committees would have granted approval well within the new time limits, although others might have taken longer. The main effect is to narrow the range of approval times.

Definition of multicentre research

Research is regarded as 'multicentre' if undertaken within the geographical boundaries of five or more local research ethics committees.

Membership of the multicentre research ethics committees

The range of experience and expertise required by a multicentre research ethics committee depends on how its role is perceived. If it is seen to be performing much the same function as a local committee, members will again need to reflect a mix of gender, age and ethnic background, drawn from throughout the region. They should include hospital medical staff, nursing staff, family doctors, other NHS professional staff and lay persons.

Alternatively, if the main function of a multicentre ethics committee is to assess the scientific validity of studies, a higher number of expert members might be required than is the case for local ethics committees. The UK committees expect to receive protocols that have already been subject to scientific assessment, although exceptions will be permitted. As a result, at least a third, but no more than half, of the membership will be lay. Experienced members of *local* research ethics committees are obvious candidates for multicentre committees and simultaneous membership of a multicentre and local research ethics committee is permissible.

Appointments to a multicentre committee

Multicentre committee members have been appointed initially for a period of two years. At the end of that time, the terms of membership will be reviewed. Either the post of chairperson or that of vice chairperson must be filled by a lay person.

Resolving differences between a researcher and the committee

It is expected that any differences of opinion between a research worker and a multicentre research ethics committee would be resolved through continuing discussions between them. Should it prove impossible to come to an agreement, referral to another multicentre research ethics committee would be permitted with the agreement of *both* the initial multicentre research ethics committee and the research worker. The advice of the second MREC will be final.

Common application forms, standards and procedures

To make life easier for the organisers of multicentre trials and to facilitate the system of cross referrals between multicentre research ethics committees, a common application form for multicentre clinical research has been developed. Local committees must accept multicentre applications on this form. A 'Supplementary Form for Local Arrangements' is also issued to local researchers to obtain additional information of relevance to local committees.

Funding of multicentre ethics committees

Funding is provided by the government. It may be considered unwise to allow the pharmaceutical industry to help fund multicentre ethics committees and training for local and multicentre committee members as this may be seen to compromise the independence of multicentre committees, despite assurances that such funding would not be tied to individual projects or paid directly to committees. On the other hand, as with local ethics committees, there may be nothing wrong in making an appropriate and realistic charge to pharmaceutical companies for the appraisal of their protocol and for protocol amendments. In 1998 the fee charged by multicentre committees for the appraisal of commercially sponsored research was £1000.

Accountability and evaluation

The multicentre research ethics committees are accountable to a senior government officer with responsibility for health. They should produce annual reports to the individual to whom they are accountable, which should be distributed to every local research ethics committee and be available for public inspection.

Responsibilities of the researcher following approval

Following approval of a project, any subsequent protocol amendments must be submitted to the multicentre ethics committee for approval before being implemented. Serious adverse events must also be reported to the committee whether or not it is believed that they are related to the study. Changes in the staff conducting the research should also be notified. The researcher is required to respond promptly to any requests from the committee for an update of the progress of the study and be willing to discuss the project with committee members.

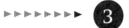

Researchers and their facilities

The researcher

Qualifications

The International Conference on Harmonisation (ICH) good clinical practice guidelines (ICH 1996, s.4.1) in common with national guidelines (Royal College of Physicians 1996, s.2.6) emphasise the importance of ensuring that the researcher is qualified to carry out the proposed research and any procedures to which patients are to be exposed. This represents a powerful argument in favour of local ethics committees whose members are likely to be familiar with the reputation of researchers and their departments, and can readily arrange to interview the researcher and view the facilities if necessary.

The principal researcher on submitting a research proposal to the ethics committee will need to give details of their qualifications and convince the committee that he or she is fully familiar with the techniques of the research and, in the case of drug trials, with the properties of the medicine being used. In order to assure the committee that there will be sufficient time to conduct and complete the study, the researcher will need to supply a list of projects currently in progress.

Any associated researchers, including the persons who will be obtaining consent from participants, must be clearly identified.

Must the researcher be medically qualified?

Article I.3 of the Declaration of Helsinki demands that biomedical research on human subjects should be under the supervision of a clinically competent medical person. Modern research is, however, increasingly initiated by biomedical scientists who are highly skilled and experienced in the problem under investigation, but who do not have clinical qualifications. Without wishing to imply that their ethical conduct is likely to be any less satisfactory, non-medically qualified researchers whose studies involve patients should ensure that those responsible for their treatment are also involved in the research. Therefore, whilst actual supervision of all research by a clinician may not be appropriate, their involvement is advisable as co-researchers and in providing medical authorisation, and being answerable to their professional colleagues or a professional conduct committee for the way the research is done.

Some research, while not involving any contact with patients, may involve the collection of confidential medical information and access to patient records. In such cases, unless the data has been effectively anonymised, the approval of a medically qualified person is also advisable.

Financial pressures

Researchers should not be under any undue pressure to recruit patients, or to retain them, against their better judgement.

Government guidance (Department of Health, 1991, s.3.15) to health authorities in the UK advises that:

> The local research ethics committee should examine any aspect of a research proposal which may influence the patient's judgement in consenting, or the researcher's judgement in his/her treatment of subjects, in such a way as to call the ethics of the research into question. Clearly any payments to subject or researcher must be considered, but it is also possible that benefits to an institution or department may raise similar ethical questions.

The ethics committee will require to see details of the financial arrangements between sponsors and researchers. Normally it is expected that payment from pharmaceutical and other commercial companies is fed into a departmental or other research fund, and they would be very concerned if it was found to be going directly into the pockets of researchers. Obviating the possibility of personal financial gain does not, in itself, however, remove the potential for undue financial pressure being exerted on researchers. They may be highly dependent on income derived from drug trials to fund their own research projects via the departmental research fund or to present their findings at an international conference.

A good initial contract between the researcher and the sponsoring company is therefore essential. Financial arrangements should allow pro rata payments for the work done and not depend on patients completing the trial or on a pre-determined number of patients having to be recruited.

Guidance from the Association of the British Pharmaceutical Industry (1994b) emphasises that:

► The payment for work carried out by an investigator in the conduct of a clinical trial should be realistic.
► All details concerning payment should be specified as part of the formal agreement, including the purposes for which staff or equipment has been funded.
► Details of the payment arrangements must be submitted to the local research ethics committee.
► Fees should be based on the hourly rates recommended by the British Medical Association for work conducted outside the National Health Service.

The General Medical Council agrees that, 'it is unethical for a doctor to accept per capita or other payments from a pharmaceutical firm in relation to a research project such as the clinical trial of a new drug *unless* the payments have been specified in a protocol which has been approved by the relevant local research ethics committee.'

For example, a pharmaceutical company in the UK, failing to achieve its recruitment targets, offered additional payments to those centres that recruited the agreed number of patients by a certain date. The offer of such payments, if they have not been approved in the original proposal, is unethical, as it might appear to act as an inducement to investigators to recruit inappropriately to the study.

Trials sponsored by pharmaceutical companies

In projects initiated not by the investigators themselves but by a pharmaceutical company or other sponsor, the ethics committee will wish to ensure that local investigators have a thorough knowledge of the projects in which they are to be involved.

For a local research ethics committee that has a modest number, say no more than six proposals to consider each month, it may be feasible to invite each local investigator to the meeting to discuss the project in person. As recognised by the Royal College of Physicians (1996, s.5.3), this is impracticable for most committees. Alternatively, some indication of the investigator's knowledge of the project may be obtained from the summary provided on the committee's standard proposal form. Ideally, therefore, the summary should be compiled by the investigator rather than by a drug company representative and should not be copied from the company's protocol.

Many pharmaceutical companies insist on completing ethics committee proposal forms on behalf of the investigators, leaving the committee with no evidence that the local investigator has even read them. A classical example is where the investigator had signed a statement to the effect that he had read the protocol and agreed with it but failed to notice that on the front page the company had given him the wrong name!

With the introduction of multicentre research ethics committees, this method of assessment may no longer be an option as the national standard application form will be completed by the sponsor.

Post-approval responsibilities
Following approval of the project, the researcher will need to:

► Notify the ethics committee immediately of any serious or unexpected adverse events irrespective of the apparent cause (ICH 1996, s.4.11.1; Royal College of Physicians, 1996, s.5.23).

► Conform to the terms of the protocol agreed with the committee, and if any amendments are necessary, gain committee approval for these before implementing them (ICH 1996, s.4.5; Royal College of Physicians, 1996, s.5.19).

► Inform the committee if additional researchers are to become involved in the trial. (Most guidelines omit to remind researchers to do this and in my experience they often forget.)

► Advise the committee if the study is suspended or terminated, giving a detailed written explanation (ICH 1996, s.4.12).

► Assist the ethics committee in the post-approval monitoring of their research should they be selected for this.

► As a courtesy, advise the committee if the study fails to get underway as a result of, for example, lack of funding.

► Remain available for contact by patients concerned about any aspect of their participation in a trial, and by family doctors or other medical staff who may need advice on how participation affects patient care outside the trial.

► Ensure that subjects are told about any information that becomes available during the trial which may be of relevance for them.

► Maintain the ability to provide appropriate medical care/follow-up of participants after the trial.

► Keep data confidential during and after the trial.

► Maintain for as long as required by national regulations, all patient files and other sources of data relating to the study, and ensure

that the facilities for archiving data remain adequate. In Britain
this period is 15 years (Royal College of Physicians 1996, s.7.47).

► As a courtesy to participants, and for their interest, consider
informing them of the results of the research in which they
participated (Royal College of Physicians 1996, s.6.39).

The facilities available

Premises and equipment

In both the UK and the USA, the availability of suitable premises
and of sterile and disposable equipment and chemicals tends to be
taken for granted, but in many parts of the world where the health
services are not so well provided for, the availability of these basic
necessities may have to be taken into account. Clearly research
cannot be allowed to proceed if participants are in danger of infection from the use of dirty needles, contaminated solutions, etc.

In proposals from UK and US hospitals, it is the availability of
items of expensive equipment that frequently has to be taken into
account rather than the basics. Care has to be taken to ensure that
the intensive use of, for example, a magnetic resonance imager or
ultrasound scanner in a research project does not result in delays
for other patients needing access to the equipment as part of their
normal clinical care. With long-term studies, care has to be taken to
ensure as far as possible that laboratory facilities, archive space
and support staff will be available for the duration of the project.

Support staff

Will additional staff be employed specially for the study or,
where inpatients are participants, is it intended to use the normal
ward staff? The requirements of the trial must not divert staff and
facilities away from the treatment of patients who are not in the
trial to the extent that trial subjects receive preferential treatment.

Suitable participants

While not to be regarded as a facility, it has to be remembered that a sufficient number of participants must be available to complete the trial. A trial which has to be abandoned before it can yield any useful results is bordering on the unethical. The researcher will need to consider the number of patients who would have been suitable for the study during the preceding year in order to ensure that the recruitment rate for the present trial will be adequate. Also, it is important to ensure that there will not be other trials in progress at the same time, thus diverting potential subjects or facilities away from the trial in hand.

4

Importance of informed consent

Article I.9 of the Declaration of Helsinki (World Medical Association 1996) states that:

> In any research on human beings, each potential subject must be adequately informed of the aims, methods, anticipated benefits and potential hazards of the study and the discomfort it may entail. They should be informed that they are at liberty to abstain from participation in the study and are free to withdraw consent to participation at any time. The physician should then obtain the subject's freely given informed consent, preferably in writing.

While the importance of informed consent is universally recognised, there is still considerable debate over exactly what informed consent is and whether consent can ever really be truly informed. As a working hypothesis, however, we will assume that informed consent is at least a partial reality.

Requirements for informed consent

The World Health Organization (WHO) guidelines (CIOMS/ WHO 1993, g.3) state that in order for informed consent to be valid, the researcher has the duty to:

▶ Communicate to the prospective subject all the information necessary for adequately informed consent.
▶ Give the prospective subject full opportunity and encouragement to ask questions.

► Exclude the possibility of unjustified deception, undue influence and intimidation.
► Seek consent only after the prospective subject has adequate knowledge of the relevant facts and of the consequences of participation, and has had sufficient opportunity to consider whether to participate.
► Obtain from each prospective subject a signed form as evidence of informed consent.

Each of these requirements is considered below in greater detail.

Provision of information

What information does the participant need in order to give informed consent?

The participant must have all of the information necessary in order to make the decision whether or not to participate. Researchers, for their part, are required to reveal the information that any reasonable person would wish to know in order to make a decision regarding his or her care. As a participant, there are many questions that might need to be asked after having had time to consider the information, as when feeling ill and anxious it may be difficult to think of the questions and even more difficult to express them. The onus, therefore, is on the researcher to supply answers to these and other questions without waiting to be asked.

As well as a verbal explanation of the study, the researcher must provide potential participants (or their relatives/carers) with a written explanation in the form of a patient or healthy volunteer information sheet (Royal College of Physicians 1996 s.7.28–7.30; 45 CFR, 46.117b; 21 CFR, 50.27). Each information sheet should preferably not exceed two pages. When the study is complex and more than two pages are required to explain all of the relevant details, consideration may be given to providing an additional summary information sheet. Potential participants can then decide from the summary outline if they are sufficiently interested in the study to proceed to the more detailed account. The more detailed account must, however, be read before consent is given.

The regulations in the USA have long stressed the importance of fully informed consent. They identify eight basic elements of informed consent plus an additional six (45 CFR, 46.116; 21 CFR, 50.25), which are optional. These still provide some of the clearest expressions of what should be included in a participant information sheet.

In the UK, the Royal College of Physicians reports on research on healthy volunteers (Royal College of Physicians 1986) and patients (Royal College of Physicians 1990b, s.7.14) and the Association of the British Pharmaceutical Industry guidelines (1988, amended 1992) advise coverage of essentially the same topics. In regard to trials sponsored by the pharmaceutical industry, the former European good clinical practice guidelines (Commission of the European Communities 1990) identified similar information needs as does the current International Conference on Harmonisation (ICH), *Guideline for Good Clinical Practice* (ICH 1996, s.4.8.10).

Further guidance on how to construct a patient information sheet in provided in Appendix 4.

The basic eight elements of informed consent

- ▶ A statement that research is being conducted, its purposes, duration and a description of the experimental procedures to be employed.
- ▶ Description of foreseeable risks and discomforts to the subject.
- ▶ Potential benefits to subjects or to others.
- ▶ Description of alternative treatments available.
- ▶ Statement regarding the extent to which research records will be kept confidential.

▶ Arrangements for compensation should the subject be harmed.

▶ Contacts for further information or redress.

▶ Statement that participation is voluntary and that the participant will not lose any treatment benefit should he or she refuse to participate or withdraw.

The additional six elements

▶ A statement that unforeseeable risks to the subject (or the fetus if the subject may become pregnant) may be involved.

▶ Circumstances in which the investigator may terminate the subject's participation.

▶ Additional costs the subject may incur.

▶ The consequences of the decision to withdraw.

▶ An agreement to provide the subject with relevant information arising during the course of the trial.

▶ Details of the numbers of subjects involved in the study.

While providing participants with a written information sheet is considered mandatory in countries like the UK and the USA, in a country with a low level of literacy, insisting on written information might severely limit the availability of participants (Cox and Macpherson 1996). The WHO guidelines do not consequently make written information an absolute requirement. However, having a written information sheet in front of participants will still help researchers to describe their projects verbally to potential recruits ensuring that all of the required information is given. Where there is only an oral presentation, US regulations require that a witness signs to confirm that this was given (45 CFR, 46.117b2; 21 CFR, 50.27b2).

In any study where there is a risk of adverse events such as fainting, participants should be advised to carry the information sheet around with them.

Helpful hints on how to write an effective information sheet and the pitfalls to avoid are provided in Appendix 4. This includes a list of 45 typical questions that can be used as a checklist to ensure that most points of likely concern to patients have been addressed and that the US (45 CFR, 46.116; 21 CFR, 50.25), UK (RCP 1990a,b) and international ICH (1996, s.4.8.10) requirements have been met.

Who should provide the information and obtain consent?

The most obvious person to obtain informed consent is the senior researcher who has designed the study. In a trial sponsored by a pharmaceutical company or other large organisation, it will be the senior researcher who although they may not have designed the study, will have been to the pre-study meetings and discussed the project with the company representatives and senior researchers at other centres.

When the senior researcher is closely involved in the participant's treatment, however, there is then the danger that the patient may feel under an obligation to participate. This danger is recognised in Article I.10 of the Declaration of Helsinki:

When obtaining informed consent for the research project the physician should be particularly cautious if the subject is in a dependent relationship to him or her or may consent under duress.

It is well known that owing to the special relationship of trust that exists between the patient and the doctor, most patients will consent to any reasonable proposal that is made to them. The Declaration goes on to state that:

in that case the informed consent should be obtained by a physician who is not engaged in the investigation and who is completely independent of the official relationship.

The highly specialised nature of much research today often makes it difficult to find a completely independent person with adequate training. In such cases, a research assistant who is involved in the project, but not directly involved with the participant's treatment, may obtain consent. When there is no alternative but for the participant's doctor to obtain consent, the doctor must ensure that the prospective participant understands that participation in the project is entirely voluntary and that the participant is not under any obligation to take part.

When the task of obtaining informed consent is delegated to a junior researcher or other member of the medical or nursing staff, care should be taken to ensure that they are conversant with the details of the project and the requirements for informed consent. Before approving an application, the ethics committee will need to know who will be obtaining consent.

Informing any other doctors who are involved with the participant's care

The Royal College of Physicians (1996, s.6.38) emphasises the importance of informing the medical staff normally responsible for the care of patients or healthy volunteers of their participation in a trial.

When other doctors are involved in the patient's treatment, they must be approached, if they are not already involved, before entering patients into a study relating to the condition being treated. A similar principle will apply when it is a family doctor who is providing treatment.

In healthy volunteer studies, it is also advisable, with the volunteers' permission, to check with their family doctor, if they have one, that they have no underlying condition that might interfere with their suitability to participate. Even when there is no medical reason for doing so, it is still a matter of courtesy to inform family doctors, to prepare them in case they are approached for advise by potential participants. Some family doctors might appreciate a copy of the patient/volunteer information sheet so that they know what their patients have been told about the project.

Full opportunity and encouragement to ask questions

The WHO guidelines (CIOMS/WHO 1993, s.3) go on to state that:

the investigator must be prepared to answer all of the subject's questions relating to the proposed research. Any restrictions of the subject's ability to ask questions and receive answers before or during the research undermines the validity of the informed consent.

The way in which information is conveyed, and when, is as important as the information itself. Presenting information in a disorganised and hurried way with too little time for consideration or discussion will make it difficult for participants to make an informed decision.

Ensuring that patients and healthy volunteers can understand is the researcher's responsibility

It is the responsibility of the researcher to ensure that participants have understood the information given to them and that the answers to their questions have also been understood. Because the ability of participants to understand depends on many factors including their intelligence, past experience, knowledge of the subject, level of anxiety, rationality, maturity and command of the language, it is necessary for researchers to adapt their presentation of the information to the participant. Different information sheets may be required, for example, when working with young children. In particular, there is a special obligation to ensure that information about risks is complete and adequately understood, and the more serious the potential risks, the greater the obligation.

Once the prospective participants have had time to read the information sheet, researchers must make themselves readily available to answer questions. Many people are reluctant to disturb doctors during the course of their work to ask what may be considered trivial questions, so it is important that researchers themselves take the lead. On more than one occasion, I have come across information sheets for children in which, in order to obtain more information about the study, they have been invited to make a peak time, long distance telephone call to the researcher. It is to be hoped that in such cases prospective participants will have the presence of mind to reverse the charges!

What if the participant is unable to comprehend the information?

When the participant's comprehension is severely limited, for example in very young children, severe handicap, advanced dementia or serious illness, the research should be discussed with a close relative or carer. That person should be given the opportunity to follow the research as it proceeds, and should be able to withdraw the participant from the study if it is in the participant's interest. Consent by third parties is discussed in more detail in Chapter 12.

To explain highly sophisticated research to very elderly patients not familiar with the modern technology, and who may have hearing and visual problems, creates a special challenge (Olde-Rikkert et al. 1997).

Consent must be freely given

Consent for medical examinations is not always given freely. The classical example is the employer who demands that prospective employees give consent to undergo a preemployment medical examination and for the company's doctor to scrutinise their medical records. The applicant gives consent only because they know that if they do not they won't get a much needed job. Obtaining consent by 'holding a gun' to someone's head in this way is unethical and would not be accepted by any medical research ethics committee if applied to potential participants in a research project. All of the guidelines agree that no one should be made to participate in a research study against their will and that great care should be taken to avoid exerting any undue influence (Belmont Report 1979, p.4; 45 CFR, 46.116; 21 CFR, 50.20; DoH 1991, s.3.5; CIOMS/WHO 1993, g.3; RCP 1996 s.7.31).

Types of persuasion to be avoided

After having been given all of the information and understood it, several factors may affect a participant's ability to decide freely whether or not to take part.

A feeling of gratitude

Patients may feel under a moral obligation to help the doctor in return for any help they have been given. Researchers therefore must ensure that patients are not taking part in research that they do not really want to, out of a feeling of obligation or as a display of gratitude.

Fear of giving offence and thereby receiving less adequate treatment

Patients should never be put in a situation where their agreement to participate derives from the feeling that not to do so would spoil their relationship with the medical staff or that they will be positively disadvantaged compared to other patients if they fail to contribute. Long-stay elderly patients and mentally ill patients are especially vulnerable in this respect, as their relationships with staff may be the only ones they have. Neither should there be any suspicion that failure to participate will result in them receiving less attention from staff. A similar principle applies to junior colleagues and students of the researcher who may fear that their career prospects will be adversely affected if they fail to volunteer.

Researchers also have an obligation to ensure that no one feels pressurised to participate in research against their real wishes. Participants must never be allowed to feel guilty or unhelpful about not wishing to be involved. This is especially important in studies that may involve such minimum input for participants that they feel it may be expected of them, but which has profound moral implications for them, which seem to have been overlooked by the researchers. An example of this is the evaluation of a new prenatal test for Down's syndrome, involving only an extra blood sample and a slightly prolonged ultrasound scan of the early fetus. Great care must be taken to make it as easy as possible for women opposed to abortion to say no, ideally by ticking the 'No' box and returning a form, without the embarrassment of having to give a face-to-face rejection to an enthusiastic researcher.

Persuasive language

As emphasised above, the use of persuasive language in patient information sheets, or indeed verbally, should be avoided.

Financial inducements

The WHO guidelines state that, 'payments to participants should not be so large or the medical services so extensive as to induce prospective subjects to participate in the research against their better judgement' (CIOMS/WHO 1993, g.4).

The Royal College of Physicians (1996, s.7.9) agrees that investigators must avoid offering patients or healthy volunteers financial inducements large enough to encourage them to agree to participate in research against their better judgement or more frequently than is advisable. Payment for risk is inappropriate, as healthy volunteers should never be exposed to more than minimal risk or patients to risks greater than those of the standard treatment. As a rough guide, it would seem reasonable if payments made to healthy volunteers on drug development trials that require them to be resident on the research wards, are set at around the average daily salary for the area. When a study involves participation for several days, in order to avoid undue pressure to continue through to the end of the study, it must be made clear to participants that if they should wish to withdraw early, they will still receive payment for the time that they have spent on the study.

In the UK, patients are rarely paid for their participation in therapeutic trials, but where patients are used as control subjects for studies unrelated to their own illness, the same rates of pay should apply as for healthy volunteers. It will have to be decided by the researcher in consultation with the ethics committee whether similar payment is also appropriate for patients involved in cost-benefits analyses where no medical benefit of the research is expected either for themselves or future patients. In regard to payment, the WHO guidelines do not distinguish between volunteers and patients.

To avoid the unthinkable situation from arising where young children, those with learning disability and others who are unable themselves to give informed consent are exploited for financial gain by their parents or guardians, a guardian consenting on their behalf should be offered no more than out-of-pocket expenses.

At a less serious level, the practice of encouraging people to return lifestyle and other non-intrusive questionnaires by offering to put their names forward for a prize draw, can probably be tolerated so long as it does not compromise confidentiality or introduce bias into the study.

The WHO guidelines go on to say that, 'all payments, reimbursements and medical services to be provided to research subjects should be approved by an ethical review committee' (CIOMS/WHO 1993, g.4). The Department of Health (1991, s.3.15) in its guidance to ethics committees in the UK shares this view.

Refund out-of-pocket expenses

The refunding of out-of-pocket expenses is not considered a financial inducement. In all cases, whether participants are volunteers or patients, reasonable travelling and other out-of-pocket expenses should be reimbursed where visits are made and where the time involved is in addition to that which would have been necessary had they not entered the study (CIOMS/WHO 1993, g.4; Royal College of Physicians 1996, s.7.11). If, as is often the case, it is necessary for someone to accompany the patient to the clinic, it would seem fair also to reimburse their travelling expenses. Participants are also likely to appreciate free refreshments, if only tea and biscuits and fruit juice, being provided at the clinic, or vouchers to exchange for refreshments, rather than having to pay what are now often city centre prices at hospital cafes out of their own pocket. Small courtesies of this kind can make participants feel that their help is appreciated, rather than that they are just being exploited as nameless research subjects.

It should be clearly stated in the information sheet that travel expenses can be claimed. A claim form should therefore be routinely given to patients without the need to suffer the embarrassment of asking for one. Investigators should also make sure that neither patients nor healthy volunteers are out-of-pocket after agreeing to participate in the research.

Other inducements
The implied promise of more attention
Other types of inducement are more difficult to avoid. Psychiatric patients are often especially vulnerable emotionally, and if participation in a research project holds out the promise of extra attention from the psychiatrist, this in itself may be a positive inducement to participate. In parts of the world where medical care is not free to patients, people may be influenced to take part in a study simply in order to obtain such care.

Unrealistically high hopes
Care should be taken never to generate unrealistically high hopes in patients about the value of a new drug. While a patient with high blood pressure is unlikely to become particularly excited about being offered yet another new antihypertensive drug to try out, unrealistically high hopes may be raised in patients and their carers in conditions such as Alzheimer's disease, where there is a serious lack of effective drug treatment (Alzheimer's Disease Society 1993). Patients may want to believe that the research will bring them some benefit, and could all too easily be induced to believe this.

Significant communication skills are also necessary to avoid raising false hopes with talk of a potentially beneficial new drug, only to dash them again on revealing that the patient is just as likely to receive a dummy drug during the trial. To avoid raising false hopes, research should always be done on the least-ill patients possible, and from the least vulnerable groups and the limitations of the new treatment carefully explained.

There are rare instances in which participation in research may bring real benefits, as when a new, effective drug can only be given to patients in a clinical trial, either because the supply is limited, or it has not yet been licensed. Benefits are, however, more likely to be perceived as real rather than actually being so. The fact that a drug is new, in short supply and expensive does not mean that it is effective!

Confidence in existing treatments and doctors should not be undermined

Pharmaceutical companies and individual researchers should never seek to undermine the patients' confidence in their existing treatment (which is perhaps manufactured by a different company) in order to recruit them to a trial of a new treatment which may turn out to be no better, or less effective, than what they are receiving already. Care should also be taken not to do this inadvertently by implying than one of the advantages of entering the trial is that their condition will be monitored more carefully than normal and they will get better treatment. If existing therapy is to be labelled 'unsatisfactory', then the criteria for this and for its withdrawal must be explicitly stated both in the proposal submitted to the ethics committee and in the patient information sheet. Similarly, confidence in their usual doctor should not be undermined by statements such as, 'If you enter the trial you will be treated by a doctor who is *specially trained* in treating your condition', which imply that their usual doctor is inadequately trained.

It is also important not to raise concerns, which patients might not otherwise have had about the standard treatment. In one proposal, the possibility of cables coming loose and staff tripping over them was mentioned as a disadvantage of the standard monitoring equipment compared with the new radio controlled monitors that patients were being asked to help test. Information of this kind only adds to the burden of anxiety in already anxious patients.

Making it easier to say 'No'

All researchers will be aware of the need to emphasise to patients that they are free to refuse to participate without giving a reason and without it affecting their future medical care. Despite this, face-to-face decisions imply a degree of persuasion and embarrassment for patients if they do not wish to participate. Ideally, if the situation allows, they should be given a simple form that they can fill in, expressing their continued interest or refusal to participate, and return in a stamped addressed envelope.

Pressure on researchers must not lead to pressure being placed on patients

Researchers are often under considerable pressure to become involved in clinical trials. This may take several forms.

Financial pressure

As discussed earlier, there is the financial pressure from commercial companies.

Peer group pressure

Many doctors are under considerable pressure from the professional groups to which they belong to put patients into trials being run by those groups. Some professional organisations take the extreme view that, in their speciality, all patients should be in a clinical trial. The researcher needs to be strong enough to resist this pressure when considering whether or not it is in the patients' best interest to continue with standard treatment rather than to encourage them to enter a trial and thereby perhaps expose them to yet more discomfort and unpleasant side-effects.

Patients should be given the choice of entering, or not, a trial, and not to be coerced into deciding between trials A, B and C. If a drug is marketed and shown to be reasonably effective with acceptable side-effects, they should be able to receive it if they wish. They should not be told that the best option on offer is a 50:50 chance of getting the drug by entering a clinical trial aimed at comparing it with something else. An obvious exception is when new conditions arise, as was the case with AIDS, where the initial absence of any standard treatment means that all treatments are at first experimental.

Medical research ethics committees need to be aware of this pressure in order to ensure that it does not result in seriously ill patients being exposed to treatments with distressing side-effects that have little prospect of providing significant benefit either now or in the future.

Can active deception ever be ethical?

Tact

There is a difference between active deception and tact. A certain amount of tact is always required in dealing with patients. When inviting patients to participate in a research project it is important not to accidentally reveal that they may have a serious condition of which they were previously unaware. In some cases, the avoidance of precise descriptions may be acceptable, such as the substitution of 'oral disease' for 'oral cancer'. In a study of a new drug for the treatment of cardiovascular disease, the statement, 'You have been selected as a potential participant in this study because you are at risk of sudden death from a heart attack', may be true, but need it be put quite so bluntly?

Incomplete disclosure is justified only if it is truly necessary to avoid alarming patients or to accomplish the goals of the research. Information about risks or discomforts must never be withheld for the purpose of enlisting the co-operation of subjects and truthful answers must always be given to direct questions about the research.

Active deception

The WHO guidelines state that deception is only permissible in studies that carry no more than minimal risk of harm (CIOMS/WHO 1993, g.3). The question of active deception is most likely to arise in psychological or social studies where awareness of the design of the study can influence the very behaviour that the researchers wish to investigate. Take as an example a study designed to compare different ways of treating anxiety. Patients are randomly allocated to one of three groups: the first group receives the standard treatment; the second receives regular home visits from a psychiatrist; while the third attends group-counselling sessions. All patients receive a quality of life questionnaire at the end of the study to compare the three treatments. If they knew that they were getting more or less treatment than other patients this could well influence their responses and invalidate the study.

Deception may also occasionally be used in a medical study to avoid influencing behaviour. An example of this is the secret inclusion of an electro-mechanical counter in an asthma inhaler in a study to determine compliance with treatment (Yeung et al. 1994).

It may be impossible to study some psychological processes without withholding information about the true object of the study or deliberately misleading the participants, but before conducting such a study, the investigator has a special responsibility (Royal College of Physicians 1996, s.7.27) to:

▶ Make sure that alternative procedures avoiding concealment or deception are not available.

▶ Ensure that deception would not inappropriately encourage patient participation.

▶ Ensure that there is an adequate plan for debriefing patients at the end of the trial and for making the results of the research available to them.

The risks of deception to the doctor–patient relationship

As well as the ethical question of whether it is right to deceive patients, there is the danger of deception affecting the long-term doctor–patient relationship.

Finding that they have been deceived could make recipients suspicious of the activities and attitudes of the medical staff who are supposed to be treating them. It is therefore very important that the reaction of participants is considered when the deception is revealed. If the deception is likely to lead to discomfort, anger or objections from the participants then it should be seen as inappropriate. In those rare cases, where incomplete disclosure can be justified, potential participants should normally be told that the research in which they are being invited to participate has certain features that will not be revealed until after they have finished taking part in it.

Participants should never be deliberately misled without extremely strong scientific or medical justification. Even then, there should be strict controls and the approval be obtained of independent advisers including the ethics committee. Care should be taken to distinguish studies in which disclosure would destroy or invalidate the research from those in which disclosure would simply inconvenience the researchers.

Allow adequate time to make a decision

As emphasised by the WHO guideline, patients must be given enough time to decide whether they are willing to consent.

Choosing the appropriate time to give information

It would clearly be unacceptable to wait until a participant was in the advanced stage of labour to invite her to participate in a study, or until a patient was on the point of having an endoscopy tube pushed down his throat before asking him if he would mind a few extra stomach biopsies being taken. Quite aside from these extreme examples, many people find it extremely difficult to read when they are anxious, or if other people are looking over their shoulder, so participants need time and space to read and digest the information sheet, and a pencil to make notes.

If at all avoidable, information should not be given at a time when the participant is unable to concentrate adequately on it, for example, during a period of anxiety about an impending operation, and certainly not in late labour. The nature of the illness itself may also impair understanding as in anxiety states or depression.

How much time to decide?

Whenever possible, the researcher should give patients and volunteers several days to decide whether or not to join a study, allowing time to get to grips with the relevant facts and consequences of participation and to talk things over with friends and relatives or their family doctor. Only after having had sufficient opportunity to consider whether or not to participate should they be allowed to sign the consent form (45 CFR, 46.116; Royal College of Physicians 1996, s.7.44).

In hospital-based studies, when participants are to be admitted from a waiting list, the researcher should have plenty of time to approach participants by letter or at an outpatient appointment. It should not normally be necessary to rush participants being recruited into an outpatient or medical practice trial into an immediate decision.

While it might seem like a good idea to post out an information sheet to patients in advance of a routine clinic appointment, care must be taken not to scare patients off attending. If this approach is taken it must be emphasised in the information sheet that no pressure will be put on them to participate should they prefer not to.

Should patients be allowed to make an immediate decision?

In studies with minimal discomfort and no foreseeable risks, or long-term consequences, participants may prefer to make an immediate decision rather than suffer the inconvenience of an extra journey to the clinic if they decide to participate. They may also be keen to get on with their treatment and not be sent away to think about it. It is not unknown, however, for a participant to express great enthusiasm for a project when first told about it, only for that enthusiasm to wane after taking the information sheet home and discussing it with relatives. They may not be keen on the participant 'being experimented on' and dissuade him or her from participating. Consent given hastily is more likely to be withdrawn later.

Where no more than minimal risk is involved and there are no conceivable ethical implications, it may occasionally be possible to justify asking for consent at the same appointment as information is supplied and for the procedure then to be carried out immediately, but the decision whether to allow this in a particular study must rest with the ethics committee. A justification for this course of action was given in a study comparing two types of marketed quick fillings for decayed primary teeth: 'It is normal practice in dentistry that some treatment, particularly if it is relatively simple such as a small restoration in a primary tooth, be carried out at the same appointment as the examination, so avoiding the need for patients and their parents to return for a second visit. In addition children (and for many of those in this study, this treatment will be their first experience of fillings) don't have time to dwell on what a further appointment might hold, nor to receive advice (usually unhelpful!) from friends as to what this might be.'

Despite the inconvenience to doctors and patients of arranging extra attendances, where more than minimal risk or discomfort is involved, patients should not be encouraged or allowed to make an immediate decision, except where a delay in initiating treatment might be dangerous.

When treatment must be initiated immediately

In some studies, the condition itself limits the time available for obtaining consent. In a comparison of different antibiotics in the treatment of severe pneumonia, or different methods of stopping a bleeding peptic ulcer, the need for treatment to be initiated as soon as possible, leaves patients with no more than a few hours in which to decide whether or not to consent. There are other cases in which the condition may be of short duration. A new ointment to ease the pain of minor soft tissue injury suffered during sporting activities, for instance, would need to be applied before the pain subsided naturally after a few hours.

A signed form as evidence of informed consent

Participants who are capable of reading the information sheet and consenting on their own behalf, should sign the consent form. It is essential, however, that researchers and ethics committee members never come to think of informed consent simply as a form that must be signed, but as a process of education that takes place between the researcher and the participant.

The American regulations require that if the participant is unable to read and therefore only an oral presentation is given, a short consent form stating that the required elements of informed consent (45 CFR, 46.116; 21 CFR, 50.27b2), as summarised on page 59, have been met must be signed by the subject, or if not, by their legally authorised representative. When this method is used, there should be a witness to the oral presentation who, along with the person obtaining consent, should sign and date a written summary of what was said.

As well as the summary, the witness to the oral presentation should also sign and date the consent form. By signing the consent form the witness attests that the written information was accurately explained to, and apparently understood by, the subject or their representative.

Essentially the same method of obtaining consent from patients in drug development trials who are unable to read has been incorporated into the ICH good clinical practice guidelines (ICH 1996, s.4.8.9).

While not an absolute requirement in other kinds of study in the UK, witnessed consent in such circumstances is seen by the Royal College of Physicians (1996 s.7.45) as a useful approach.

The institutional review board may waive the requirement for a signed consent form if: (1) the principal risk of harm to the subject would be a breach of confidentiality resulting from the signed form; or (2) the research presents no more than minimal risk of harm and involves procedures for which consent would not be required outside research (45 CFR, 46.117c). There are also obviously emergency situations in which it may not be feasible to obtain a signed consent form (Office for Protection from Research Risks 1996).

In studies which involve no physical risk to the participant, such as making use of spare blood samples, it may be tempting to make do with verbal consent only, but written consent should normally be obtained. Only if there are no ethical issues involved in the use of the spare blood/tissue, and there is no possibility of new results being linked to the participant, is verbal consent acceptable in such cases (Chapter 13). One of the few situations in which verbal consent is acceptable is when a new diagnostic test is being evaluated. If, for example, a swab has been taken for detection of genital *Chlamydia* infection by the standard test as part of routine clinical care and it is desired to take an extra swab to evaluate a new test for the same microorganism, as no new information of relevance to the patient can be generated, and only a minor procedure is involved, verbal consent would be adequate.

US regulations expect a combined information sheet/consent form (45 CFR, 46.117b1). In the UK, however, the consent form is often separate from the information sheet. See Appendix 5 for a specimen consent form based on that recommended by the Royal College of Physicians (1990 s.7.20). This consent form necessitates responding to individual questions to encourage prospective subjects to reflect, as each question is ticked in turn, on whether they have actually read the information sheet. Also it gives the participant an opportunity to ask questions and discuss the study, to receive satisfactory answers to all of their questions, to receive enough information, and to understand the voluntary nature of participation. Investigators should check the consent forms carefully to ensure that participants have indicted by their ticks against individual questions that they are satisfied with the information provided. The participant's signature at the bottom of the form should not be accepted if they have failed to respond to any of the questions, or responded in the negative, until the problem has been resolved to the participant's satisfaction. The American regulations emphasise that consent forms must not have any wording appended that seeks to undermine the subject's legal rights in the event of injury resulting from the study.

The consent form should be witnessed. This can normally be done by the person obtaining consent. If, however, the patient has intellectual or language difficulties in understanding or is extremely distressed, but still deemed capable of giving informed consent, the signature of an *independent* witness in required (Royal College of Physicians 1996 s. 7.0). If the patient is incapable of giving informed consent on their own behalf, the consent form should be signed by a relative or carer.

It is not specified in the UK guidelines that the information sheet itself (if separate from the consent form) should be signed by the subject, but doing so would provide further evidence that it has been read, and should be encouraged.

In questionnaire studies that include questions which are intrusive and may cause distress, the study must be explained, and written consent obtained, prior to issuing the questionnaire. Where the questions are innocuous, as for instance with most dietary questionnaires, the fact that the subject returns the questionnaire may be taken as implied consent.

Where should the signed consent forms be kept?

Signed consent forms should be kept by the researcher in the research records so that they are readily available for scrutiny by ethics committee monitors. When the participants are patients, a copy of the consent form, along with a copy of the information sheet, should be placed in the hospital case notes, so that other doctors responsible for the patients' treatment are aware of the participation and what it involves. In the UK, records should be kept for a minimum of 15 years (Royal College of Physicians 1996, s.7.47). Patients should also be given a copy of the consent form and information sheet to keep (45 CFR, 46.117b2).

Informed consent for tests to find suitable participants

The main government and professional guidelines offer no advice on this. There will be many occasions when it will not be certain whether a participant fulfils the criteria for joining a study until admitted to hospital and further tests have been done. Can preliminary tests be done with limited consent? In many cases these tests will be part of standard care and only observation will be required to determine suitability. When, however, the tests required to confirm eligibility are additional to those required for normal clinical care, the investigator should obtain informed consent before performing them. When nothing more invasive than a few extra millilitres of blood or a urine sample is required, or even an additional biopsy during a routine endoscopy, the question arises whether it is justifiable to trouble sick participants with reading an information sheet for a study that may increase their anxiety when, in all likelihood, they will not be suitable participants anyway.

In such situations, it may be considered acceptable to provide a preliminary information sheet and consent form that simply asks patients if they would consider letting the researcher perform the test to see if they would be eligible for a research project related to their illness. It should be made clear that they are under no obligation to agree to the preliminary test, and that doing so does not commit them to taking part in the main study later on. If found to be suitable they would then be given further details to help them decide whether to participate. This approach would not be acceptable if the preliminary test carried more than minimal risk or if there was any possibility of it yielding information with serious implications for the patient.

Eligibility for a study may also depend on what treatment the patient receives following admission. If the initial treatment is outside the control of the researcher, or required due to circumstances, procedures may be carried out, or drugs given, that would interfere with the study and render the patient unsuitable.

The local research ethics committee will need to consider each case carefully in deciding what dispensations, if any, are permissible in order to avoid inconveniencing large numbers of patients. Is it acceptable to wait until patients are established to be suitable participants before approaching them and consequently reducing the time they have available to reflect on the proposal before needing to give consent? Each study will need to be considered on its merits.

Keen to participate but unwilling or unable to sign a consent form

Occasionally it may happen that patients are keen to participate in a research project but unwilling to sign a consent form. This situation may arise due to concerns about confidentiality, as for example in HIV or following abortions. As indicated, in such cases US regulations allow the institutional review board to waive the requirement for the investigator to obtain a signed consent form

(45CFR, 46.117c1). It is, however, preferable if the support of participants is gained by a careful explanation of the mechanisms in place to ensure confidentiality.

Research on patients without informed consent

The ultimate in deception is to involve patients in research projects without their knowledge. Can this ever be ethically acceptable?

While the Declaration of Helsinki strongly emphasises the importance of informed consent, it does recognise in Article II.5 that there may be rare situations in which it can be waived:

> If the physician considers it essential not to obtain informed consent, the specific reasons for this proposal should be stated in the experimental protocol for transmission to the independent committee.

When the patient's consent is impossible to obtain

In research on conditions that result in emergency admissions of unconscious patients, the luxury of time does not exist and a rapid decision may be necessary if the patient is to be entered into the trial. Examples are a comparison of different methods of resuscitation following a heart attack, or the treatment of stroke where a new drug designed to limit the extent of damage in the brain would need to be administered within a few hours of onset. Studies of this kind where it is impossible to obtain the patients' consent or that of their relatives in time for treatment to be initiated may represent a special case, where the otherwise universal requirement for informed consent may be waived by an ethics committee if, after seeking expert advice, it is convinced of the scientific validity and potential benefit of the trial. In such cases, as soon as patients recover sufficiently or their relatives can be found, their consent should be sought (Office for Protection from Research Risks 1996; Royal College of Physicians 1996, s.8.18).

The issues associated with obtaining informed consent in emergency situations and from young children and those with learning disability are discussed in more detail in Chapter 12.

Studies not impacting on individual patients

When the process of obtaining informed consent would involve the researcher in a great deal of extra work for something which is likely to be of little or no concern to the patient, the temptation exists to go ahead without the patient's knowledge. Epidemiological and database studies often produce this temptation. These are discussed in more detail in Chapter 15.

When it may be more unethical to tell patients

In some studies, consideration has to be given to whether patients are more likely to be harmed by being told the reason for the research than by it being conducted without their knowledge (Tobias and Souhami 1993). In an epidemiological study aimed at determining whether persons with certain characteristics are at greater risk of dying of cardiovascular disease than the general population, some people might become extremely alarmed at the suggestion, even if it were as yet unproved. The ethics committee has to consider each such study on its merits. The potential harm that might arise from a breach of confidentiality has to be balanced against the harm that might result from creating unnecessary anxiety.

Except in studies where patients are too ill to give consent or, at the other end of the spectrum, where the research is confined to the scrutiny of anonymised patient records or the use of spare blood and other tissue without impacting on participants, there are very few instances where it would be ethically uncontroversial to conduct research on patients or volunteers without their informed consent. Even studies on spare tissue, as discussed in Chapter 13, frequently pose serious ethical issues.

The right to withdraw consent

The right of patients to refuse to enter a study has been fully discussed; the right to withdraw consent after having entered is of equal importance. Despite best attempts to provide all of the relevant information, the participant may not have fully realised what was involved in the study before entering it, and may now be having second thoughts.

Investigators must ensure that participants are fully aware of the fact that they have the right to withdraw from a research project at any time and for whatever reason (45 CFR, 46.116 a8; 21 CFR, 50.25a8; Royal College of Physicians 1996, s.1.16 & 7.38). Each subject information sheet and consent form should include a statement similar to the following:

> We stress that participation in this study is entirely voluntary. You are free to decline to take part and you can withdraw from the study at any time without having to give a reason. This would not affect your present or future medical care, or your relationship with the staff looking after you.

The right of withdrawal must also be made clear verbally. In the case of participants receiving payment, such as healthy volunteers in drug development trials, they must understand that payment for the effort put in does not depend on completing the study.

In post-approval monitoring of research, local research ethics committees will wish to ensure that the right to withdraw is being exercised. While they will be concerned if too many participants are withdrawing from projects, and curious to know why, they will equally be concerned if hardly anyone ever withdraws.

Avoiding undue pressure to stay in a trial

It is important, therefore, to ensure that participants are not placed under undue pressure to remain in a trial against their will. How could this happen? In the case of a very rare condition where suitable patients are few and far between, it is easy to envisage a situation arising where a researcher might be reluctant to let go, especially if the consequent fall in numbers would undermine the statistical validity of the results obtained with the remaining patients.

As already discussed, there are also financial pressures. Research departments are paid substantial sums for the research they do for drug companies. If remuneration depends on participants completing the study, a researcher could be influenced to try to persuade them to continue. Steps can be taken to reduce the risk of the temptation arising in the first place. Funding arrangements between drug companies and researchers should allow for payment on a per visit basis so that if the patient drops out after the first visit, the doctor at least gets paid for the effort already put in.

No responsible researcher would place undue pressure on a patient to stay in a trial if the patient's health was at risk. However, he or she might be tempted if the patient wished to withdraw for reasons which, although real enough to the patient, seem trivial to the researcher, like not wanting any more needle pricks or to put up with minor side-effects such as drowsiness or constipation.

Can participants ever be denied the right to withdraw?

Can there ever be an exception to the rule that the participant's right to withdraw should be clearly stated in the participant information sheet? It may be justifiable to omit this statement if withdrawal might prove harmful once a patient has embarked on the study. The possibility of such a non-withdrawal situation arising should be acknowledged by the researcher on submitting the project to the ethics committee for its consideration. The committee must then decide whether the special considerations justify waiving the usual right to withdraw.

Long-term monitoring of new procedures

In the development of new procedures where the long-term effects are not known it may be essential to monitor patients for several years after they have undergone the procedure. The use of pig's hearts for transplantation serves as an example. As the risk of transmission of diseases from pigs to humans needs to be established, it will be essential to subject patients to a battery of tests at regular intervals in the years following the operation.

In such circumstances it may be acceptable to make it a condition of participation in a trial that the patient does not withdraw from the subsequent monitoring, although there is likely to be little that can be done if he subsequently decides to do so.

The point of no return

Surgical procedures, in particular, may have a point of no return. For example, in a comparison of two methods of hip replacement, once the procedure has been done by one method, it cannot be undone and repeated by the other.

The researcher's right to withdraw patients

Where appropriate, it should also be made clear to patients in the patient information sheet that the researcher has the right to withdraw patients from the study if, for whatever reason, it is considered in their best interests to do so (45 CFR, 46.116b2; 21 CFR, 50.25b2).

The researcher must establish before the start of the research the withdrawal criteria for patients, and this be communicated to the ethics committee. Typically patients will need to be withdrawn if they:

- ► Have a significant worsening of their condition.
- ► Have an adverse event unacceptable to the patient or doctor.
- ► Require other treatment non compliant with study requirements.
- ► Become pregnant.
- ► Develop a serious unrelated illness which may interfere with the study.
- ► Fail to co-operate adequately with the conduct of the study.
- ► If information about unacceptable side-effects of the drug or procedure becomes available from other centres.
- ► The sponsors decide, for whatever reason, to cancel the study.

There will be additional withdrawal criteria specific to particular studies. For example, in a trial of a new antihypertensive drug this would be the elevation of a patient's blood pressure above a certain predetermined level, or in a trial of a new lipid-lowering drug, a rise in lipid levels above what is acceptable. Alternative treatment could then be implemented or, if the trials were placebo controlled, those in the placebo group put on active treatment.

It is appropriate to conclude a chapter on informed consent by quoting from Article I. 3 of the Declaration of Helsinki:

> The responsibility for the human subject must always rest with a medically qualified person and never rest on the subject of the research, even though the subject has given his or her consent.

5

Evaluating risks and benefits

The Declaration of Helsinki (World Medical Association 1996) forbids the exposure of research participants to unnecessary risks. Article I.4 demands that:

> the importance of the objective is in proportion to the inherent risk to the subject.

Do the potential benefits justify the risks?

This is the key question which researchers and ethics committees must address before a research project involving patients or healthy volunteers can be approved (45 CFR, 46.111a2; CIOMS/WHO 1993, g.2; Royal College of Physicians 1996, s.71).

The prime responsibility of a medical research ethics committee is to protect participants from harm. While no committee will wish to hold up potentially valuable research, they must ensure that individuals participating in the research are never exposed to unacceptable risk and that every possible step has been taken to reduce risks to the absolute minimum necessary to fulfil the purposes of the research (45 CFR, 46.111a1). The balancing of risks and benefits is an activity common to all kinds of clinical intervention, but in the treatment situation it is the patient who stands to benefit directly. In research, although the participant may sometimes benefit, the benefits are more likely to accrue to future patients and society as a whole in terms of a better understanding of how diseases arise, their prevention and treatment. As a result there is an even greater awareness of the need for patients to be kept fully informed of any risks involved and for these risks to be minimised.

Assessing risks

How much risk should the patient be allowed to accept?

A certain amount of risk is inevitable. If you invite enough people to attend for screening, there will be a significant possibility of someone becoming involved in a road accident on the way to the clinic!

Most research involves the possibility of some risk to the participant, ranging from fatigue at having to fill in a never-ending questionnaire to long-term physical harm arising from an unexpected serious adverse drug reaction. So long as the risks are clearly explained and fully understood, should it not then be up to the participants themselves to decide whether or not to take part in the research? The answer must be, 'No!' While this might seem to be depriving people of their freedom of choice, we have to be aware that there may be some individuals willing to expose themselves to risks over and above what it is reasonable to expect of anyone. For example, they might have a special reason for wishing to help overcome an illness that they do not wish others – their children for instance – to suffer from in the same way as themselves.

Psychological factors may also affect a patient's ability to decide. An extreme example would be patients with depressive delusions who consent to research that they consider unpleasant and hazardous because they believe they are unworthy and should be punished! More commonly, pressurised by a sense of gratitude to the doctors, or fear (hopefully unfounded) of not getting the best treatment if they refuse to participate, some patients might agree to expose themselves to risks which, as healthy volunteers, they would not consider acceptable.

These are just a few of the reasons why it is unwise to let the decision as to what is an acceptable risk lie solely with the participants. This is in addition to the initial problem of ensuring that participants fully understand the risks involved.

The role of the medical research ethics committee

Medical research ethics committees provide a necessary safeguard for participants, allowing an independent assessment of whether it is ethical to invite them to expose themselves to the risks associated with a particular piece of research. If in the judgement of the committee it is not ethical to do so, this judgement must take priority over that of the patient. On the other hand, an assessment by the committee that the risks associated with the project are acceptable in principle must never be allowed to override or belittle the patients' assessment of the risk as being unacceptable to them personally. An ethics committee might consider the risk of having a tooth extracted under general anaesthesia acceptable, but the patient with a relative who had died in a dentist's chair might consider otherwise. In both cases, the more cautious assessment carries ethical priority.

Care also has to be taken to ensure that the correct emphasis is being placed on the risks. There is a tendency for less emphasis to be placed on the risks and side-effects of a drug when it is first being developed for the market, than when it has become the old treatment against which a new improved drug 'with fewer side-effects' is being compared.

What risks should be revealed to patients?

Should all risks and side-effects, no matter how rare, be stated? There is no consensus on this matter. The World Health

Organization (WHO) guidelines (CIOMS/WHO 1993, s.2) take the balanced view that although it may not be feasible in complex research projects to inform prospective participants fully about every possible risk, they must be informed of all risks that a reasonable person would consider important in making a decision about whether or not to participate.

There is clearly a need to be sensible in the reporting of risks. There could be a power cut in the middle of an operation and the emergency generator that was supposed to take over might not have worked! However, while in the UK and the USA the risk of such an eventuality is currently so remote that no one would seriously consider including it, in parts of the world with a less reliable electricity supply, it might not be possible to brush aside the risk so lightly. Risks are locality specific, depending on the facilities and skills available in the centres concerned, and are factors that need to be assessed by *local* ethics committees.

In standard clinical practice it is rare for the doctor to go into a detailed description of everything which could conceivably go wrong. It should again be emphasised, however, that the ethics of standard clinical practice are governed by the principle that the patient's interests should always come first, whereas in research it is frequently not the present patient or healthy volunteer who stands to benefit but future generations of patients.

How much risk is acceptable from the procedure or treatment?

Basic non-therapeutic research

For basic non-therapeutic research involving healthy volunteers or patients where no benefit to the participants is anticipated, it is generally agreed that they should be exposed to no more than *minimal risk*. This may be defined as a risk of injury or death that is no more than that encountered in daily life. This is obviously a difficult thing to quantify as some people's daily lives involve more risk than others. For example, a construction worker's daily life is likely to be considerably more hazardous than that of an office worker. We clearly need to err on the side of caution.

Another frequently used definition is that the risk should be no greater than that of travelling by a scheduled airline but, as heavy traffic makes walking more dangerous than flying, the minimal risk level may then be exceeded even before the patient reaches the clinic.

Therapeutic research

For therapeutic research where the patient may personally benefit from the treatment, for example, when two antibiotics are being compared, *minimal risk* might be defined differently as that which is no greater than the risk of the care that they would be receiving were they not in the trial.

The risks of depriving patients of standard treatment

A complication arises in trials where a new drug is being compared with a placebo. In placebo controlled studies some patients may be receiving no effective treatment, making it necessary to take into account the risks of no treatment, as well as those associated with the new drug. The ethics of placebo controlled trials are considered in more detail in Chapter 10.

High risk with trivial consequences, or low risk with devastating consequences

In discussing risks a distinction must be made between adverse events, of which there is a high risk but which would only have minor consequences, and serious adverse events, of which there is a low risk but would have serious consequences if they occurred. Many different kinds of harm have to be taken into account, including psychological harm, physical harm, social harm, and financial harm.

In certain kinds of study, notably those identifying the genetic origin of a disease, the risks of research may extend beyond the individual subjects to their families. Also, society at large or special groups of subjects in society may sometimes be affected.

Should we concern ourselves with the risks to society?

The risks to which society or the environment may be exposed as a result of a treatment are not always given consideration by researchers or medical research ethics committees. Examples are the disposal of radioactive waste arising from a new form of radiotherapy, or (before they started to be phased out) the damage to the ozone layer caused by propellants used in certain inhaled treatments for asthma. Neither is the researcher nor ethics committee likely to concern themself with the risks of, for example, a new high-tech treatment deflecting limited health service resources away from less glamorous preventative strategies that might have brought more benefit in the long-term.

This situation is, however, changing. In the area of animal to human transplantation, the possibility of introducing animal viruses associated with the transplanted organ both into the recipient and into the wider human population is a risk that must be taken into account when considering whether or not a study should be approved. If there are serious environmental or resource implications of the research, an ethics committee will be expected to draw them to the attention of the researcher, and ask how they are to be dealt with and whether they can be justified.

Minimising the risks

In any study, the most important consideration must always be the health and safety of the participants. The researcher must be prepared to halt a subject's participation at any time if it is felt that continued participation would be detrimental to their health (World Medical Association 1996, article III 3).

Risks can never be entirely eliminated, but they should be

reduced to what is absolutely necessary to achieve the research objective (45 CFR, 46.111a1). The following guidelines will help to ensure that risks are kept as low as possible.

Good exclusion criteria for subjects

In drug development studies, it is important to ensure that patients who may be especially sensitive to the harmful effects of a new drug are excluded. For the testing of new drugs on healthy volunteers this means ensuring that the volunteers are indeed in reasonable health. This will usually necessitate contacting their family doctor and conducting a pre-study medical examination including an electrocardiogram and blood pressure measurement to exclude volunteers suffering from heart disease or high blood pressure. Women who are pregnant should normally be excluded. If women of childbearing age take part, pregnancy tests should be performed before and at intervals during the study, and participants warned about the need for adequate contraception.

Good criteria for contra indications

Investigators must establish in advance what the criteria will be for withdrawing participants from the study. In a placebo-controlled trial of a new anti-hypertensive drug this will mean clearly establishing before the study commences at what blood pressure level patients will be withdrawn and provided with alternative treatment to get their blood pressure down.

Proper monitoring of research subjects

Adequate monitoring of patients is essential if the risks associated with a clinical trial are to be reduced to an absolute minimum. In the example above, regular monitoring of patients would be necessary to ensure that any rise in blood pressure was detected before it reached a potentially dangerous level. The ethics committee would need to assure itself that the frequency of visits to the clinic for blood pressure checks were adequate.

Rapid response to and reporting of adverse events

Although routine monitoring of a participant's heartbeat in the trial of a new drug may sound reassuring, it is meaningless unless there is someone in constant attendance to observe the monitor, and who has the skills to initiate treatment in the event of anything going wrong. In any study, whether for example, of new drugs or procedures or exercise tolerance, where a serious adverse event may occur, however unlikely, clinical staff trained in resuscitation techniques must always immediately be available.

Immediate code breaking in the event of adverse events in blind or double-blind trials

In pharmaceutical company trials in which neither the patient nor the researcher knows who is receiving the active drug or placebo it is essential that, should anything go wrong, the researcher would be able to break the code with the minimum of delay to find out what treatment the patient was receiving.

Long-term follow-up

Patients should not be abandoned at the end of a trial if there is the remotest possibility of long-term side-effects, whether physical or psychological. This necessitates ongoing medical and psychological support and counselling where necessary.

The well-being of the researcher and support staff

In considering the ethics of a research proposal it is sometimes necessary to consider the well-being of the researchers as well as that of the patients.

Emotional exhaustion

Let us consider a study designed by a department of obstetrics to find out whether their bereavement programmes actually help parents to come to terms with the loss of their newborn infants. All the parents who agree to be involved in the study are invited to take part in an in-depth interview three months after the death of their infant, usually in their own homes.

Being in receipt of powerful emotions will be exhausting and no doubt distressing for any researcher involved in this kind of project. If visiting families involves extensive travel this could create a certain risk to the researcher if their concentration were impaired by emotions arising from the interview. It is therefore essential that mechanisms be in place to ensure that the interviewer is adequately supported during this period. Support persons should be nominated to ensure that the well-being of the interviewer is safeguarded.

Handling difficult patients

Within the hospital environment certain types of research can also create problems for staff. Taking severely mentally disturbed patients off their medication in the run up to a trial, for example, may make it extremely difficult for the nursing staff to manage such patients. They may be exposed to considerable distress or even the risk of injury.

Fetal tissue

In studies employing fetal tissue, some members of staff may be extremely distressed at the prospect of handling this material. It is essential that, like patients, they should have the right to refuse to participate without their career prospects being affected.

When research is likely to be emotionally taxing for the staff involved, due consideration must be given to its effect on them. Research ethics committees need to ensure that the design of the proposals coming before them adequately take into account the interests of vulnerable staff as well as of patients.

Determining benefits

Benefits are notoriously difficult to assess, especially when, as is usually the case, no one knows for certain whether the research will be of benefit or not. If they did, there would often be little point in doing it. It is usually the potential benefits that may or not happen which are being assessed, rather than actual benefits.

Basic research

In basic biomedical research, the anticipated benefits may be very long term and unlikely ever to be reaped by the participants, who may in any case be healthy volunteers. Initially encouraging lines of investigation frequently lead nowhere, and fail to benefit anyone. The more basic the research, the less certainty there is that any benefit will ever accrue from it.

Therapeutic research

The potential benefits are usually more clearly defined in therapeutic research, although the precise degree and probability of benefit is often difficult to predict. Benefits may be somewhat easier to assess when small-scale trials have already shown the drug to be of value so giving a good idea of what to expect in a larger scale trial.

What kind of benefits should be included in the equation?
Only the additional *benefit of the new treatment should be taken into account*

In assessing the potential benefits of a new drug or procedure, it is the *additional* benefits over and above those normally achieved by the current standard treatment (45 CFR, 46.111a2) that should be considered. In a trial of a new antibiotic to combat a serious infection, saving the patient's life cannot be claimed as a benefit of the new antibiotic if a dozen other antibiotics currently on the market could have done that equally effectively. If, however, the new antibiotic had a lower incidence of unpleasant side-effects, this could justifiably be classed as a benefit. Complicating the assessment of benefit is the appearance of strains of bacteria that are resistant to some of the standard antibiotics and that having new antibiotics in reserve may indeed turn out in the future to be potentially life saving.

Duplication of existing drugs

The potential benefit that may arise from duplicating existing drugs is always difficult to assess. Is any overall benefit really likely to result from the development of yet another H2 antagonist for the treatment of ulcers or yet another anti-hypertensive drug? It is rare for ethics committees to turn down research proposals because they consider that there are already enough drugs of the kind under investigation on the market. The pharmaceutical companies will always point out that they are attempting to develop drugs with fewer side-effects, or side-effects that may make them more acceptable to a larger number of patients, or drugs that work by a different mechanism and may be effective in patients who do not respond satisfactorily to the current treatment.

Should psychological benefit be included?

Should psychological benefit arising from the feeling that 'something is being done' for the participant be included in the ethics committee's deliberations of benefits? Only if it can be established that the extra attention is not at the expense of patients not in the study.

Benefits not to be included

As well as better treatment for patients, other potential benefits of research include development of the researchers' expertise, attraction of prestigious research funding to a department and enhancement of the reputation of the research institution. Benefits of this kind though real should be *excluded* from the risk-benefit analysis.

Research on participants without direct medical benefit?

Many people may well take the view that to be ethical, research on patients and volunteers must aim to yield some medical, emotional or social benefit for participants. But are there any circumstances in which research not aimed at directly benefiting patients either now or in the future can be justified?

Research aimed at saving money – cost-benefit analyses

Is it acceptable to invite participants to take part in research, the sole aim of which is to find ways of saving money? Increasing demands on the limited budget of a health service may lead to an increase in the amount of research being carried out purely for financial reasons. Although 'research' to establish the most cost effective method of treating patients may not benefit those who participate in it, there is the argument that it may enable much needed funds to be released for use elsewhere in the health service, for example, to buy new equipment or employ more nurses (or more accountants?). Most of the published guidelines remain silent on the issue.

The following is a suggested set of cost-benefit analysis guidelines:

▶ Research carried out for financial reasons should never involve more than minimal risk or discomfort for patients. If it did, it would be unethical even if conducted with their full consent.
▶ A cost-benefit analysis should never be the primary aim of research carried out on children or those with learning disability.
▶ Patients must be made fully aware of the true aims of the study.

- ▶ Participation in a cost-benefit analysis should not be the only way of getting the better treatment.
- ▶ Cost-benefit analyses should not be financed out of funds otherwise destined for 'real' research.

A typical example of a cost-benefit analysis

In order to illustrate some of the ethical issues surrounding cost-benefit analyses, an example of one such finance-based research project is considered. It concerns two antibiotics – one old, one new. The old antibiotic has been in use for many years to treat acute infections, but some strains of bacteria have become resistant to it and one patient in three now fails to respond. A new antibiotic has recently been developed which is nearly 100 per cent effective in treating this kind of infection, but it is expensive.

A cost-benefit analysis is therefore devised to compare the cost of using the two antibiotics. Patients are randomly allocated to one of two groups. The first group will be given the old antibiotic first, and the one in three who fail to respond will then be given the new antibiotic. The second group will receive the new antibiotic from the start.

The aim is to determine which treatment is cheaper overall. The increased cost of the new antibiotic is to be balanced against the cost of the extra stay in hospital for patients who fail to respond to the old antibiotic.

As it has already been established that the new antibiotic is more effective than the old, is it not unethical to repeat the study just to determine the relative cost, thereby inflicting a longer period of illness on some of the participants? Should not all of the patients receive the new treatment regardless of cost as part of their standard clinical care? Ideally, the answer to both questions should be, 'Yes!'. But it cannot be assumed that a medical research ethics committee would reject this proposal, or others like it, before it reached the patient as many members will see virtue in ensuring value for money.

The ultimate decision whether to participate is therefore likely to be left to the patient.

Researchers must make patients aware of the true aims of the study

Patients can only make an informed decision about whether to participate if the researcher makes it absolutely clear that the study is a cost-benefit analysis and not real medical research. The title of the patient information sheet should make this immediately apparent as well as being emphasised again within the text of the sheet so that patients can be left in no doubt about the motive behind the research. This will allow those with a genuine interest in ensuring that treatments represent value for money to join the study, while those unwilling to suffer inconvenience or a possible prolongation of their illness for the sake of saving the health service money are free to decline.

When participation in a cost-benefit analysis is the only way of getting the better treatment

A serious ethical dilemma arises when patients who decline to participate then have to make do with the older, cheaper, less effective drug, and are not even given the 50:50 chance of receiving the better drug granted to those who enter the study. Finding themselves in this situation, patients may consent purely to give themselves a chance of receiving the new drug, not because they approve of the cost-benefit analysis.

Financial research should not be funded out of budgets for 'real' research

Of major concern is the possibility that finance-based research may direct research funds and staff resources away from pure medical research. Research ethics committees and indeed participants themselves should always ask where the funding is coming from. It is undesirable for finance-based research to be financed out of medical research budgets. Another budget, the most obvious being the one that is most likely to benefit from improved cost-effectiveness of treatment, should be tapped for this purpose. It should also fund the additional staff time required to carry out the project, leaving existing staff free to participate in pure medical research.

More complex examples of cost-benefit analysis

The antibiotic study above is a comparatively straightforward example with cost cutting the primary aim. Most studies involving cost-benefit analysis are more complex than this, often including genuine efforts to compare the effectiveness of different methods of treatment along with the cost element. This leaves the ethics committee and the patient wondering which takes priority and how to apportion the risks and benefits.

Take as an example, a study aimed at determining whether it is feasible for patients to treat themselves with intravenous antibiotics at home rather than relying on hospital medical staff or community nurses. Whilst cost cutting is a significant motive, if it proved to be feasible, it could also be perceived as an advantage to those patients who do not wish to have to remain in hospital for a moment longer than necessary or those patients whose journey to hospital is too difficult. If the patient is exposed to additional risk, the ethics are difficult to assess, as it is impossible to say to what extent the risks are being run to see if money can be saved or for the sake of the increased convenience of patients.

There are many areas of medicine where a treatment that has been in use for many years is expensive and no one is certain whether it really works in all patients. Finding a way of predicting which patients are most likely to benefit would not only save money, but save patients wasting their time and being exposed to any risks associated with the ineffective treatment. Such research is therefore potentially extremely valuable.

Studies of this kind, which include a genuine attempt to benefit patients, are likely to be looked upon more kindly by patients than those where the aim is purely to save money.

Environmental effects

Another kind of study, which may be of no direct medical benefit to patients themselves, is one designed to reduce the harmful effects of treatment on the environment. A good example of this arises from the phasing out of chorofluorocarbons (CFCs).

Chlorofluorocarbons

Because of the damage they cause to the ozone layer, CFC propellants are being phased out of use in most of their applications. Major suppliers worldwide have announced their intention to discontinue production and by the early 1990s many nations had adopted laws or resolutions limiting, or eliminating altogether, their use over the next few years.

Patients become involved because CFCs feature as the propellant in inhalers used in the treatment of asthma and other respiratory illnesses. Faced with the impending ban, pharmaceutical companies are attempting to develop inhalers containing alternative propellants that are believed not to harm the environment. As a result, clinical trials need to be conducted to assess whether the inhalers with the new propellant (which may also require a modified formulation of the drug) are as safe and effective as the current CFC inhalers. So long as patients are made fully aware of the reason for testing the new inhaler, are not exposed to any undue risks and understand that there is no direct benefit to themselves, but consent out of concern for the environment, there will usually be no ethical objection to such studies.

As medical use accounts for only a tiny proportion of the total consumption of CFCs, should serious problems be encountered in developing new propellants, it is perhaps not too much to hope that inhalers would be exempted for a number of years until satisfactory alternatives were found.

Other studies without medical benefit

An example of a less obvious way of how hospital patients can be involved in non-medical studies, which does not fall within the previous two categories, is as follows. Forensic pathologists wish to obtain a more reliable means of estimating for how long murder victims and others have been dead – referred to as the post-mortem interval. There is a promising group of proteins that break down slowly after death which may provide a means of estimating the post-mortem interval. Rather than removing tissue from patients who have just died with its inherent problems of obtaining consent from relatives, the researchers plan to investigate the rate of break-down of the different proteins on biopsies taken from the mouths of patients undergoing oral surgery. This study uses patients simply because they are a captive audience, there being no scientific reason why healthy volunteers could not be used instead.

If patients are being approached simply because it is feared that no healthy volunteers would come forward for the procedure, then the patients are being unfairly exploited, and the study is unethical and should not be approved. A better reason for using patients would be if the equipment and staff are readily available for performing the procedure, whereas to do it on healthy volunteers might involve considerable extra time and expense. If subjects needed to be anaesthetised, this would not be acceptable for healthy volunteers, and it would therefore be necessary to recruit patients who were already being anaesthetised as part of their normal clinical care. In non-medical studies of this kind, it is essential that participants are made fully aware of the aims of the research and that it can hold no benefit either for themselves or future patients. They must not be made to feel under the least obligation to participate.

Research ethics committees that carry out post-approval monitoring may wish to put such studies near the top their list, and invite patients to be interviewed or to complete a questionnaire to determine whether they fully understood what was involved and the aims of the study before agreeing to participate.

6

Acceptable research procedures

Non-invasive procedures

Many research projects involve the patient in nothing more invasive than having a few extra millilitres of blood drawn over and above that required for clinical management, or a probe passed gently across the surface of the skin.

Procedures of this kind, which at the time of writing, appear to carry no known risks include:

- ▶ Microlightguide spectrophotometry – a technique used to measure the amount of oxygen in the blood passing through the skin, performed by lightly scanning over the surface of the skin with a lightguide probe. It takes less than a minute for each scan.
- ▶ Laser Doppler imaging – a technique which involves scanning a harmless light beam over the surface of the skin enabling blood flow to be determined from changes in the reflected light.
- ▶ Thermography – a camera is positioned over the bed where the patient is lying and an image is taken of the blood flow in the deeper layers of the skin.

All of the above scans are painless and nothing is placed into the skin. They have a wide range of potential uses, from measuring changes in the blood flow in response to the administration of therapeutic drugs to learning more about the changes that occur in the breast following radiotherapy, or to determining the best point for limb amputation.

- Ultrasound scanning – with such diverse applications as observing the fetus developing in the womb, to measuring bone density in the ankle to estimate the risk of osteoporosis. Although traditionally regarded as a safe procedure, it would be a wise precaution to avoid excessive exposure of the early fetus to ultrasound.
- Electrocardiogram and blood pressure measurements.
- This list can be extended by adding procedures from the list of: 'research activities which may be reviewed through the expedited review procedure', produced by the Office for Protection from Research Risks in the United States (see page 30), most of which, apart from venepuncture, fit into this category.

There are, however, other procedures employed in research that are invasive and themselves carry an element of risk.

Ionising radiation

Research involving the administration of ionising radiation to patients and volunteers has been conducted for many years often with inadequate awareness of, or concerns for, the potential risks involved. The US Advisory Committee on Human Radiation Experiments set up by President Clinton in 1994, found that there had been serious human rights abuses in radiation experiments done in the 1950s and 1960s (Faden 1996), while claims of similar abuses have recently been investigated in the UK (Nicholson 1997b).

●●●●● **Summary of guidance in the UK on the use of radiation in research without direct benefit to the participants (National Radiological Protection Board, 1988)**

- The radiation should only be applied by properly qualified persons and with the approval of the local research ethics committee.
- A certificate of authorisation should be obtained.
- There should be no other means of achieving the same objective.
- The dose should be kept as low as consistent with the objective and

normally no higher than that in category III (defined in the guidance notes).

► Participants should have freely given their informed consent.

► Participants should normally be over 50 years. Younger persons should only be used if the research is specific to their age group. If the research is with children under 16, the dose should be within category I (defined in the guidance notes).

► Pregnant women should not be included unless the project specifically concerns pregnancy.

► The number of subjects should be kept to a minimum to avoid unnecessary exposure.

► The total effective dose should not exceed 50 mSv in a year. Volunteers should therefore be asked if they have taken part in any other projects within a year.

► Records of administered doses should be kept and be available to volunteers.

► Persons receiving a dose of more than 15 mSv in a year from their occupation should not normally be accepted as participants.

Ethics committees should not approve a study involving ionising radiation without prior approval from an appropriate radiation safety committee where such a committee exists.

Invasive procedures

Invasive procedures possibly acceptable for research purposes alone
Blood sampling

A low risk invasive procedure like taking a sample of blood from a vein in the arm is acceptable in competent adults with their permission, so long as the amount and frequency are reasonable. The amount taken should not normally exceed in any three-month period that which it would be permissible to donate for transfusion. To avoid extra needle pricks, it should be arranged with clinical colleagues, whenever possible, to draw extra blood for research into a syringe at the same time as it is being taken for clinical tests.

To avoid frequent needle pricks, when a large number of samples are required, an indwelling catheter should be used. Blood sampling from an artery such as the brachial artery in the arm, potentially carries more risk and should only be done when really necessary and by those properly trained in the procedure. It should not be done in children (British Paediatric Association 1992, p.9). Researchers should avoid exposing young children, seriously ill patients, and persons with learning disability to extra needle pricks, or any other form of blood sampling, except when absolutely necessary.

Nasogastric intubation

The insertion of a tube through the nose into the stomach is routine in patients after an operation and, while causing some discomfort, might be considered acceptable if done purely for research purposes in healthy volunteers. For example, for sampling stomach fluids to assess the effectiveness of a new drug in reducing acid secretion.

Additional endoscopies and biopsies of the digestive tract

Studies on the digestive tract, such as those comparing the rate of ulcer healing in response to different antibiotics and antacids, typically require endoscopy and biopsies of the gut wall to enable the diagnosis to be confirmed and to follow the patient's response to treatment. So long as they are performed with the latest techniques and in skilled hands, an ethics committee may accept additional endoscopies and biopsies in such studies. Similarly, flexible sigmoidoscopy may be permissible for examining the structure of the wall of the large bowel in, for example, patients on different nasogastric feeds.

Skin biopsies

The taking of small skin or muscle biopsies from inconspicuous areas of the body may also be permissible in basic biochemical studies of skin conditions. In all cases, the researcher must fully inform the potential subjects of exactly what the procedure involves, the potential risks, discomforts and side-effects, such as, in the case of a skin biopsy, the size and location of a subsequent scar, and the risk of infection. Naturally, subjects must not be pressurised into participating.

Invasive procedures not justified for research purposes alone

Major procedures that carry more than minimal risk are only justified if there is significant potential benefit for the participant. It is unlikely that procedures such as lung or liver biopsy, bone marrow removal from the breast bone or cardiac catheterisation could ever be justified for research purposes alone, either on children (British Paediatric Association 1992, p.9) or adults. This applies even though the patient may be eager to participate. It may, however, be considered acceptable to make use of such procedures to obtain information in a research project when they are *already being conducted* to diagnose or treat the patient's condition.

While it is unlikely, for example, that a medical research ethics committee would countenance the insertion of a needle into the spine specifically to remove spinal fluid for research purposes, it may be willing to agree to the removal of a small volume of spinal fluid if a needle is already in place for a valid clinical purpose, such as administering an epidural anaesthetic. But only, of course, with the patient's written informed consent.

The choice of invasive procedures for diagnosis or treatment must not be influenced by the demands of the research unless the procedure itself is being studied.

Before approving a project, the medical research ethics committee will need to be satisfied that the choice of procedure will not be influenced by the demands of the research. Additional invasive procedures must never be performed, ostensibly 'for clinical reasons' but primarily because they provide the opportunity to pursue the research. In the case of the epidural anaesthesia, for example, patients should not be influenced to choose this method of anaesthesia simply so that the researcher can get the spinal fluid required.

So that the decision as to which treatment procedures are employed is seen to be independent of the requirements of the research, the participants should preferably be patients of a doctor not involved in the research rather than patients of the researcher. In practice, this separation may not always be feasible.

Any procedure can be dangerous in unskilled hands

As well as its inherent dangers, the risk of a procedure is also highly dependent on how, where and by whom it is performed. Withdrawing blood from a vein in the arm is virtually risk free in UK or USA hospitals where single-use, disposable needles and syringes are always used. This procedure, however, would be potentially lethal in a situation where the same equipment was used over and over again with inadequate sterilisation in between. Similarly endoscopy and biopsy of the stomach carry minimal risk when performed by an experienced doctor with access to up-to-date facilities, but in unskilled hands could have unfortunate consequences. As emphasised in Chapter 3, the medical research ethics committee is under an obligation to establish that researchers have the experience and facilities available to conduct their proposed research safely before approval is given.

Low risk procedures can become high risk in seriously ill patients

Dentists are often reluctant to offer treatment to patients with serious heart disease. This emphasises the point that everyday, low risk procedures may carry significant risks in unfit patients. With some procedures, such as endoscopy and flexible sigmoidoscopy, risks, in skilled hands, can be virtually eliminated by excluding from the research very elderly patients and those with severe disease of the heart and circulatory system.

Invasive research procedures in routine clinical use elsewhere

The argument is sometimes advanced that although the invasive procedure that is intended to be used in the research project is not part of standard clinical practice in the hospital concerned, it is routine for similar patients in a centre or centres elsewhere. It does not follow, however, that because an invasive procedure is accepted as standard clinical practice that it is acceptable purely for research purposes. Higher levels of risk may be acceptable if the patient stands to benefit directly than if the procedure is being done purely for research, where the benefit, if any, is likely to be to patients in the future. Moreover, local researchers may be less experienced in the procedure than doctors in centres where it is carried out routinely.

An invasive research procedure which may be turned to therapeutic benefit

The situation becomes more complex when an invasive procedure, which it is proposed to carry out during a research project, but which is not routinely carried out on such patients, can be taken advantage of to directly benefit them. An example of this would be arthroscopy, a procedure that involves inserting a broad needle into the knee joint under local anaesthetic. While not acceptable for research purposes alone, the procedure may become more acceptable if the surgeon takes the opportunity to remove debris from the joint at the same time, thus providing patients with some relief from pain for a few weeks.

Cardiologists sometimes wish to use invasive procedures in

research aimed at understanding more about the functioning of the heart, but as already stated, highly invasive procedures are not acceptable for research purposes alone. The researcher may argue that although the procedure would not normally be carried out in his department on such patients, the information so obtained as part of a research project would be of value in diagnosing and treating the individual patient.

The medical research ethics committee will need to take great care in assessing the validity of any such claims, seeking expert advise where necessary from outside the committee.

Expert knowledge may be necessary to assess the risks of invasive procedures

Some invasive procedures are relatively easy for the patient or ethics committee member to comprehend, but others are more taxing. Below is a description of an invasive procedure from an actual research proposal:

> a hemostatic vascular sheath will be inserted into the left subclavian vein and through this a pulmonary flotation catheter is inserted (while you are lying relaxed we will introduce a tube to monitor the heart pressure into a blood vessel under the left collar bone). This carries a small risk of pneumothorax (air appearing in the lining of the lung), haemothorax (blood in the lining of the lung), pulmonary infarction (damage to lung tissue), inadvertent puncture of the subclavian artery (main blood vessel to arm) or thoracic duct (lymph drainage vessel in chest), pulmonary artery trauma (damage to the lung blood vessel), knotting of the catheter, infections and transient arrhythmias (abnormal heart rhythm).

How can either the patient or a non-specialist member of a medical research ethics committee be expected (even with the bracketed translations) to assess the risk from such a procedure? If there is no cardiovascular specialist on the committee, it will be necessary to seek the advice of an outside specialist as to the significance of the risks.

Plans for dealing with emergencies arising during invasive procedures

In assessing the acceptability of a procedure, the ethics committee will need to know what plans are in place to deal with an emergency, even if the chance of one arising is remote. In some studies it will be necessary to ensure that a member of staff skilled in cardiopulmonary resuscitation is present throughout the procedure.

When the procedure itself is only part of the research

Once the procedure is done, that may be the full extent of the patient's involvement. In other cases, the procedure may form part of a wider study in which the patient will be required to take a new drug, or to come off current treatment. These may carry additional risks, all of which will need to be carefully taken into account in assessing the proposal, as emphasised in Chapter 5.

What should be the time interval between studies?

There is no simple answer to this question, as the extent of the involvement of patients differs markedly between studies. In drug development studies it is generally accepted that the gap between the end of a patient's participation in one study and entering another should be at least three months. As well as being essential for the safety of the patient, a significant interval may also be necessary to avoid invalidating the results of the second trial. If this rule, however, were to be universally applied to all research studies beyond those involving the administration of medicines, it would severely restrict the availability of potential participants and limit the research that could be done.

In the absence of official guidance on the subject I have devised a set of guidelines as follows:

► There should be at least a three-month gap between participation in studies involving the administration of drugs.
► There should be at least a three-month gap between studies in which significant quantities of blood are removed.

► With studies involving a lot of time and effort on behalf of patients above that required for standard treatment, with multiple early morning clinic visits, for example, a three-month gap will also be appropriate.

► When a study involves patients in additional exposure to procedures known to carry an element of risk, such as moderate/high dose X rays; they must be excluded from studies that employ the same procedure for as long as recommended by the appropriate safety experts.

► When a study involves exposing patients to procedures to which excessive exposure *might be suspected* to carry an element of risk, such as additional ultrasound scanning of the fetus, patients should not be invited to take part in another study involving the use of the same procedures within three months.

► In studies that involve patients in no additional risk, or significant amounts of extra effort, time or discomfort, the three-month rule may be waived. Typical examples are studies that involve a single blood test, the completion of a non-intrusive questionnaire or access to medical records.

► Whenever the three-month rule is not to be observed the intention and reason for not doing so should be stated in the application to the medical research ethics committee.

► Heads of departments, in consultation with each other, should ensure that studies conducted by their staff are properly co-ordinated, to avoid the same patients being pounced on by several different groups of researchers within a few hours of being admitted to hospital.

One group particularly susceptible to over-researching are maternity patients. Although many of the studies are likely to involve nothing more than completing a questionnaire or an extra blood sample, care should be taken not to unduly pester women in what many see as an extremely vulnerable situation (AIMS 1997).

Other patient groups in high demand as research subjects include those with asthma, diabetes, high blood pressure and learning disability. Care must be taken to ensure that patients visiting their family doctor or an outpatient clinic on a regular basis do not get so heartily sick of being asked to participate in yet another study each time they attend that they give up attending, with a possible detrimental effect to their health.

Simultaneous participation in two or more studies

Would it ever be acceptable for there to be no interval at all between studies, with patients taking part in two or more at the same time?

This is not necessarily so alarming as it may sound. Take the example of two research groups each wishing to obtain a 5 ml sample of blood from the same type of patient for different purposes. It would seem more sensible to obtain 10 ml of blood from 50 patients and, split it, rather than 5 ml from 100 patients.

Epidemiological studies may go on for years. When participation means no more than having to complete a simple questionnaire, or to donate a small blood sample once a year, it would be unrealistic to prohibit participation in another study during this period. So long as participation in more than one project does not place patients or healthy volunteers in any additional risk, discomfort or emotional distress it may be considered acceptable.

Conversely, in drug trials, a patient's or volunteer's involvement in two studies at the same time is likely to invalidate the results of both studies, and is something which researchers are keen to avoid. To reduce the temptation for volunteers in financial difficulty to offer themselves as subjects too often is a frequently quoted reason for ensuring that the level of remuneration for research participants remains low.

Prior to recruiting patients or healthy volunteers to more than one study at a time, or within three months of the end of a previous study, the intention and reason for doing so must be communicated to the medical research ethics committee and their approval obtained.

7

Confidentiality

Article I.6 of the Declaration of Helsinki (World Medical Association 1996) states:

> Every precaution should be taken to respect the privacy of the subject and to minimise the impact of the study on the subject's physical and mental integrity and on the personality of the subject.

Respect for the privacy of the subject is demonstrated by obtaining their permission before releasing any confidential information about them and by taking all reasonable efforts to minimise the risk of a breach of confidentiality during a study.

Preserving the confidentiality of patients or volunteers is as important in research as in standard clinical care. When the researcher is also the patient's doctor or a member of the team providing treatment and the research data is kept in the researcher's office, the same rules of confidentiality will apply as in normal clinical practice. Then the only new issue of confidentiality likely to be raised by the research is that of whether and to whom the findings should be disclosed.

Additional issues of confidentiality arise, however, when the researcher is neither the doctor of the patient who is to be studied nor working in the same department or organisation. This is a typical feature of epidemiological studies.

Accessing medical records and data bases

Researchers wishing to identify patients with a particular illness for recruitment to their study may write to family doctors or appropriate consultants within the geographical area of interest, asking for the names and addresses of patients with the condition, or alternatively request access to hospital medical records.

This raises the issue of acceptability. Is it acceptable for family doctors or hospitals to supply information about their patients to researchers, or does this represent a serious breach of patient confidentiality? It is important to recognise that personal medical records serve as the starting point for a great deal of valuable clinical and epidemiological research, and that care should be taken not to introduce constraints that discourage access to them by bona fide researchers.

Obtaining patients' permission for access to medical records

In epidemiological studies involving the scrutiny of thousands of computerised records, it may be impracticable to seek the permission of every patient and may even be unethical if it causes large numbers of unaffected individuals needless anxiety. The Royal College of Physicians (1996, s.8.24) advises that so long as the same strict code of confidentiality is observed when medical records are used for research purposes as in standard clinical practice, it may not always be necessary to ask the patient's permission first. The College takes the view that in studies which would not otherwise involve contact with patients, access to medical records is acceptable without their individual consent provided that the doctor responsible for their care or, if this is not practicable, the medical officer or other appropriate official in the institution that holds the data, gives written permission (Royal College of Physicians 1996, appendix B). It also recommends that the principal recipient of the information should be a senior professional person, such as a consultant medical practitioner or senior family doctor, who is subject to an effective disciplinary code enforced by their professional body over any breach of confidentiality, for example by suspension from practice in a serious case.

Is approval by a medical research ethics committee required?

If individual consent is not to be obtained, the World Health Organizations (WHO) epidemiological guidelines (CIOMS/WHO 1993, g.2) state that 'an investigator who proposes *not* to seek informed consent has the obligation to explain to the ethical review committee how the study would be ethical in its absence'. Despite the implication of the CIOMS/WHO guidance that ethical review is indeed required in research requiring access to medical records, the Royal College of Physicians (1996, s.6.23) does not regard ethical review as always essential if no patient contact is involved.

To enhance confidentiality in studies requiring access to medical records, the following precautions are recommended:

▶ Any application for access to medical records should state the reason for which the records are needed and what steps will be taken to keep them confidential.

▶ The names and status of the person or persons who will have access to the records must be provided, and they should each sign a declaration of confidentiality.

▶ The approval should have a specified time limit for the research project rather than giving indefinite access, which might result in the records being used for purposes not in the original agreement.

▶ When data is transferred from the main records to a research database, patients should, whenever possible, be identified only by code.

Ethics committees, like the guidelines, are likely to differ in their view as to whether research that simply involves access to medical records with no patient contact or implications needs to be submitted to them for scrutiny. Researchers are therefore advised to contact their local medical research ethics committee for advice before proceeding with the research.

Contacting patients

When *direct contact* with patients with a particular condition is involved, the consensus view is that this does indeed require individual consent and ethical review (Royal College of Physicians 1996, appendix B).

The Royal College of Physicians (1996, s.8.27) advises that the initial contact should be made through the family doctor or consultant. It may be possible, with the approval of the ethics committee, to waive this requirement and allow direct access to medical records and direct contact by a researcher not involved in the patient's treatment if the researcher is, nevertheless, employed in the same department. Ideally the doctor (or dentist, ophthalmologist, etc.) should give the patient a simple form to sign consenting to their details being passed on to the research group, but emphasising that this does not place them under any obligation to participate. If this approach is not taken and doctors divulge names to researchers without permission, or researchers extract a list of names from a computerised database, some patients on being contacted may well consider that a serious breach of confidentiality has taken place and issue a formal complaint to the health authority.

Letters are a potential serious source of breaches of confidentiality. They may be delivered to the wrong or an old address or otherwise fall into the wrong hands. Imagine the trauma of a child opening her parent's mail only to find out that her mother or father is suffering from a serious illness of which she was previously unaware. Or a student may have left instructions with a flatmate to open his mail while he is travelling abroad little realising that confidential medical information would be revealed.

It is also extremely important to check that patients are still alive before trying to contact them. Receiving a letter inviting a dead relative to attend a clinic or participate in a research trial can be very distressing for some people, and is a frequent source of complaint against the health service.

For these reasons, as advised by the Royal College of Physicians, whenever feasible, family doctors or consultants who know the patients personally and are aware of their individual circumstances should make the initial contact. Opportunistic contact as patients attend for clinic appointments, or a confidential telephone call, might be considered preferable to a letter with its potential for misdirection.

Computerised medical records may be used to generate random lists of individuals of a specified sex or age group for sending out general questionnaires. When the questionnaire does not label the individual as having a particular condition, the questions are non-intrusive and it is clear that the subject is under no obligation to complete it, it may be acceptable to distribute it directly without using the patient's family doctor as an intermediary. Return of the questionnaire will be taken as implied consent (Royal College of Physicians 1996, s.7.50).

Computerised case registers and other databases

A research database

On both sides of the Atlantic, confidential information about patients is routinely entered onto computer databases in hospitals and in medical practices and is transmitted to government health departments. As well as information required for hospital management purposes, standard codes indicating the patient's diagnosis and any operations or procedures performed is often included. Although they now serve as a useful source of information in many epidemiological and audit studies, such databases were typically set up as a management and billing tool and are not the direct responsibility of the medical research ethics committee. The setting up of a case register of patients with a particular illness purely for research purposes does, however, raise issues of medical research ethics, so let us now consider the issues surrounding the process.

Why a patient case register?

The reasons for setting up a case register include:

- ▶ Finding out how common a disease is.
- ▶ Assessing the accuracy of its diagnosis.
- ▶ Obtaining an improved understanding of the epidemiology of the disease.
- ▶ Maintaining a list of patients, carers and doctors who may be willing to participate in basic research or clinical trials of new treatments.

In setting up a research database, every effort should be made at the design stage to exclude non-health service organisations, such as insurance companies and employers, from gaining access to the confidential information. Although precise official guidance on the subject appears to be lacking, it would seem prudent when dealing with psychiatric or serious physical conditions, where disclosure of confidential information could have an effect on the patient's livelihood or social standing, for informed consent to be obtained before entering these details on a case register.

The setting up of a register of patients with a serious condition should, therefore, involve the following steps:

- ▶ The researcher should ask the doctor, who is the source of the information about patients with the condition, to make the first approach to the patients, informing them that there is a researcher wishing to set up a database of patients with their condition. The doctor should then ask their permission to pass on their name and address to the researcher. Even when researchers have obtained the names and addresses of patients directly from a standard database they should, when feasible, obtain the doctors' agreement and help in making the initial contact.

► Having given permission for the researcher to approach them, patients should be provided with a simple information sheet and asked to sign a consent form if they agree to be included on the register.

► Once the diagnosis is established by scrutinising patients' case notes, the information must be anonymised by deleting their names, addresses and dates of birth and allocating a code number before registration on the database (CIOMS/WHO 1991, g.26). Holding a simple list of names and addresses corresponding to the code number in a locked cupboard remote from the main register will enable the code to be broken by the principal researcher if required.

► Confidentiality will be improved if the name of the patient's family doctor or consultant is omitted from the file and they too are identified only by code number.

The exclusion of confidential patient information is especially important if the computer is attached to a network.

Medical audit

Audit studies also may involve the creation of new databases with the transfer of data of varying degrees of sensitivity from management databases. The local medical research ethics committee should always be contacted for advice on whether it is necessary first to ask the patients' permission. In some large scale audit and research studies involving data of comparatively low sensitivity it may not be feasible. A key question is whether the risk of revealing confidential information by contacting patients is greater than if it were recorded without their knowledge.

There are a growing number of audit studies in which patient details are transferred by doctors to researchers co-ordinating the audit via the Internet. Whenever the Internet or a local network is involved it cannot be emphasised too strongly that patients must be identified by a code, which is identifiable only by the doctors concerned. It should go without saying that the code must *not* include the patient's date of birth and that no patient details should be given that could lead to them being identified by hackers illegally entering the system.

It has to be recognised that the high level of suspicion prevalent in some parts of the world surrounding the keeping of personal information on computer databases may render an activity taken for granted in the UK and the USA totally out of the question, even with the patients' permission.

The UK Data Protection Act

Most countries have some type of data protection designed to protect *data subjects* (i.e., people about whom data is held on computer). The following is a discussion of how the UK Data Protection Act (1984) operates. It is advisable for readers in other countries to check the details of their own legislation, although the description of the UK legislation may provide tips on what to look for.

In the UK, the holding of personal data on computer or in other electronic form is governed by the Data Protection Act of 1984. This Act applies to all kinds of data held on computer, not specifically health service data, but it does not apply to paper records, for which other codes of confidentiality are available (Department of Health 1996a). The Act, however, was revised in 1998 (for 1999 implementation) to cover some manual records.

Who should register?

Any individual or organisation holding personal data on a computer, other than pure mailing lists, is required to register with the Data Protection Registrar. On registering, the *data user*, who may be an individual or an organisation, must state the *purposes* for which the data is being held. This is usually done by selecting from a standard list provided by the Registrar. For each stated *purpose*, the *data holder* must then state to whom he may wish to *disclose* the information. This again usually involves selecting from a standard list.

The issue of whether an individual researcher or the employing research institution should be registered in respect of a particular research activity depends on who exercises overall control of the contents and use of the personal data concerned. If the researcher is employed by a hospital to conduct research in a particular area then even if he or she has considerable discretion regarding the approach to be taken and in determining what personal data are held in connection with the research, the researcher is merely acting on behalf of the employer. This distinction is not always clear. A university may employ someone largely because of their distinguished research record in a particular area, and the individual concerned may well bring on-going personal research with them. In such circumstances it may, in practice, be difficult to draw a distinction between research that is done on behalf of the employer (the university) and research which is essentially private. If in doubt in a particular case, the advice of the Data Protection Registrar should be sought.

The eight principles of the UK Data Protection Act are each discussed below in regard to how information is used for medical research (Data Protection Register 1989).

1   Information should be obtained and processed fairly and lawfully

When *data users*, who in our case are likely to be medical researchers, request information about potential participants, either from themselves or from others, they should make sure that they appreciate what it will be used for and that they are not misled as to its purpose, or who will have access to it.

The first principle of the Act, however, gives a special dispensation for personal data held for historical, statistical or research purposes. Information will not be regarded as obtained unfairly merely because its use for those purposes was not disclosed when the information was obtained from the *data subject*. This means that a researcher, who uses for research, data that was originally collected for clinical or management purposes is not contravening the Act, even if patients have never been told that information about them may be used in this way.

Also the first principle states that there should be no unfair pressure used to obtain the information – no unjustified threats should be made or inducements offered. Neither should participants be led to believe that they must supply the information and that failure to do so might disadvantage them. This aspect of the first principle closely conforms with the requirements for obtaining freely given informed consent discussed in Chapter 4.

2 Personal Data should be held only for one or more specified and lawful purposes

In registering with the Data Protection Registrar, the *data user* must specify for what purposes the data will be used. If the *data user* wishes to use information for a purpose other than that specified, an amendment to the original registration should be made before doing so. As well as being registered, purposes for which the data will be used must of course be lawful.

3 Data must be used only for those purposes and only be disclosed to those people described in the register entry

In registering with the Data Protection Registrar, *data users* must also specify all of the persons or organisations to which they may wish to *disclose* the data.

When they first register, in order to ensure that they do not subsequently break the terms of their registration, health authorities and hospitals tend to err on the side of caution and include in their register entry every organisation and type of individual they could conceivably wish to disclose information to, now or in the future. With these all-embracing registrations, it is often difficult to find anyone to whom they are *not* allowed to disclose personal information under the terms of the Act. As a result, the UK Data Protection Act offers less protection to patients in respect of confidentiality than might have been hoped. Fortunately, so far as health care staff are concerned, the same rules of confidentiality apply to data held in electronic form as that kept on paper, so protection of confidentiality does not depend on the Act alone.

4 Personal data must be adequate, relevant and not excessive in relation to the purpose for which they are held

This principle aims to ensure that the personal data held for a particular purpose are sufficient, but not more than sufficient for that purpose.

Thus researchers wishing to study patients with a specific illness, should not have on their computer a copy of the complete hospital database containing the medical details of hundreds of thousands of patients who do not have the illness being studied. Neither should the files in their possession include personal information about patients irrelevant to the condition being studied. In requesting data, researchers should specify to those in charge of the computer systems exactly what information is required so that only relevant data will be supplied.

When contact with patients is not required, prior removal at source of all patient identifiers is an alternative approach.

5 Personal data shall be accurate and, where necessary, kept up to date

Inaccuracies in computer held data must be avoided if they are likely to cause damage or distress to the data subject or others. Central hospital databases are constantly being updated, but an independent research database, or an extract of data from the central database, may not be. One typical result is the attempt to contact patients who have died with consequent distress to relatives. To reduce the risk of this happening, care should be taken, where appropriate, to ensure that information on databases is kept up to date.

If it is found that incorrect data has been accidentally passed on to a third party, every attempt should be made to make them aware of the inaccuracies at the earliest opportunity.

6 Personal data should be held no longer than is necessary for the registered purpose

The Registrar's guidelines state that:

> To comply with this principle, data users will need to review their personal data regularly and to delete the information which is no longer required for their purposes.

This would seem to conflict with research guidelines that state that information should be held for 15 years after the end of a clinical trial. The Act states, however, that personal data which are held for historical, statistical or research purposes and which are not used in a way which is likely to cause distress or damage to any *data subject* may be kept indefinitely. They must of course, be kept secure.

7 Individuals have the right to access data held about themselves and where appropriate to have the data corrected or deleted

In general, everyone has a right to know and to receive a print out of what information is held on computer about him or her. There is, again, a special provision in regard to data held for research purposes, which effectively means that the *data user* does not have to reveal it. It is, nevertheless, a matter of courtesy to provide participants of research studies with this information if they should request it, and this should be considered normal practice, so long as it is not likely to cause participants damage or distress. To supply information in one case does not, under the Act, mean that researchers have relinquished the right not to do so in other cases if they should be swamped with requests as a result perhaps of media attention.

8   Appropriate security measures shall be taken against unauthorised access to, or alteration, disclosure or destruction of personal data and against its accidental loss

Unauthorised access and disclosure

Researchers must ensure that the data being used are held securely. They should ensure that personal data can be accessed, altered, disclosed or destroyed only by authorised people. All personal files should be password protected, the password being known only to those authorised and it should be changed regularly. Care should be taken to ensure that staff are aware of their responsibilities regarding confidentiality. Proper consideration should be given to the integrity of staff who will have access to the personal data. If an employee is found to be unreliable, or is dismissed, it is the researcher's responsibility to ensure that that employee's authority to access personal data is immediately withdrawn.

Most of the precautions that need to be taken are self evident, but easily overlooked. Computers should not be left switched on in a place where passers-by can read data off the screens or printers, or in a room to which anyone can gain access when the *data user* is not present. Care should be taken to clean tapes and discs before being re-used rather than writing data over the old when there is the possibility of the old personal data remaining to reach someone who is not authorised to read it. Printed material containing information extracted from the computer files should be kept in a locked filing cabinet or disposed of securely by shredding.

Accidental or deliberate damage

Every effort should be taken to reduce the risk of loss due to burglary, fire, viruses, other malicious damage, equipment failure or spilled coffee. Keeping office doors locked and chaining computers to desks, frequently changing passwords to restrict access and running virus checks with an up-to-date version of anti-virus software are some of the standard precautions that should be implemented *before* loss occurs rather than, as tends to be the case, *after* it occurs.

The *data user* is responsible under the Act for ensuring that regular back-ups of important information are kept on floppy disk or other electronic media, in case, despite all of the precautions, loss still occurs. This is particularly important if participants could be harmed by the loss of computerised information relevant to their participation in a clinical trial, such as details of drugs given and their response to them. Back-up copies should be kept as secure as the original data, ideally in a fireproof safe remote from the main site.

The lack of appropriate security measures as well as contravention of any of these eight principles may lead to a *data subject* being entitled to claim compensation from the *data user* for any damage resulting from the disclosure or loss of personal information.

While the UK Data Protection Act mainly applies to records held in an electronic form, it is expected that researchers will wish to pay equal regard to the security of their paper records.

Disclosure of personal information derived from research

Research results must not be disclosed without participants' consent

Before beginning to recruit participants, the researcher will need to consider carefully if there is any possibility that the research could throw up, perhaps inadvertently as a result of a routine screening test, any information relating to the patient's health of which they, their relatives or family doctor should be informed. If so, in accord with the normal principles of informed consent, patients should be told before consenting to the research who exactly the results may be disclosed to.

Also, will the participant be told the results of any tests? Will their family doctor be informed? Who else will have access to their case notes – e.g. drug company representatives, members of a monitoring team from the ethics committee?

Genetic studies and insurance companies

Genetic studies raise special issues of confidentiality arising from the fact that if an illness in an individual is found to be due to a specific genetic mutation, it can have implications for other family members who may be carriers of the mutation. As they may develop the illness themselves in later life, or pass it on to their children, does the doctor have a duty to tell the relatives about the genetic abnormality affecting their family, even if this means breaching the confidentiality of the original patient? This emphasises the importance of obtaining the participant's informed consent to disclosure prior to entering the study to avoid this situation arising in the first place. The special ethical issues raised by genetic studies are discussed in more detail in Chapter 16.

There is currently concern among researchers in the UK that the widespread publicity given to the potential interest of insurance companies in confidential genetic information might influence the willingness of patients to take part in valuable genetic research (Daniel 1997). The all-embracing registrations made by employing research institutions, hospitals or universities usually mean that disclosures could be made to insurance companies without a criminal breach of the Data Protection Act. The absence of such a sanction could well weaken public confidence. Researchers should therefore be encouraged to approach their employing authority with a view to seeking to revise the relevant register entries to expressly provide that no disclosures of personal data held for research purposes can be made unless the express informed consent of the individual data subjects has been obtained. This would have the effect of making it a criminal offence to make a non-consensual disclosure. (One of the main reasons for a hospital to include insurance companies as a disclosure category is for the purpose of, for example, defending negligence claims.) Where a hospital released only aggregate data they would not be making a disclosure of personal data.

Leaving aside the question of registration, it would seem quite clear that a non-consensual release of personal data would breach the common law duty of confidentiality owed to individual patients/data subjects. This would then involve unlawful processing in breach of the first principle of the Data Protection Act. A breach of a principle is not of itself a criminal offence. However, the Registrar may issue a formal enforcement notice requiring the data user to amend their practices in order to conform to the requirements of the principles. Where a hospital, university or researcher continued to make non-consensual disclosures of personal data without any clear legal basis and in breach of an enforcement notice, that data user would commit a criminal offence.

Where a disclosure is made with the individual data subject's consent then, by virtue of section 34(6)(a) of the Data Protection Act, this would not involve a criminal offence even if the disclosure is not listed in the data user's entry. A disclosure of personal data can be made without a breach of the Act where there is clear informed consent of the individual data subject concerned.

Subsequent further disclosure by those to whom personalised computerised information has been disclosed

An anomaly arises when a researcher discloses information to a family doctor who may then pass on the information to an insurance company or any other organisation. If the doctor does not computerise the information concerned then it may not constitute personal data according to the Act. The Act was revised in 1998 to cover some manual records. It should, however, be perfectly possible to address this issue as a matter of formal contract so that if, for example, a family doctor disclosed information to an insurance company or other organisation, not only would they be very likely to be in breach of their own responsibilities in respect of the duty of confidentiality owed to patients (and presumably therefore put themselves at risk of having formal action taken against them by the General Medical Council) but would be in breach of a contractual agreement anyway. Registration merely serves to ensure that a particular disclosure will not involve a criminal breach of the 1984 Data Protection Act. It does not make them immune from legal action. A researcher making a disclosure of personal data to a family doctor would have to be satisfied that the data subject concerned was aware of, and had consented to, such a disclosure in the first place.

The use of video/audio recordings

Participants should be told exactly what the recordings will be used for and great care taken to ensure that only those persons or groups for whom the participant has given permission have access to them (British Sociological Society, 1993). The Royal College of Physicians (1996, s.8.1) takes the view that it is good practice to give participants the opportunity to review the recording after it has been made, so that they may withdraw consent and have the material erased if they wish. The ethics committee should require a statement from the researcher regarding arrangements for the ultimate erasure of confidential recordings. When audio or video recordings are being used for teaching purposes, to preserve the confidentiality of the original participants, consideration should be given to re-recording, using 'actors' to speak the words of the patients, omitting any personal identifiers.

Avoiding inadvertent breaches of confidentiality

The golden rule is that before medical records or tissue samples are removed from the premises of those directly responsible for the patients' clinical care, the names and addresses should be erased and the patients identified only by code number.

As well as the possibility of identification through paper or electronic records, the possibility of direct breaches of confidentiality through personal contact should not be overlooked. Researchers should take care to ensure that confidentiality is not compromised by such oversights as allowing subjects to be photographed during a press visit to a new research facility or by allowing normal controls to attend a clinic at the same time as patients. If, for instance, the physical and intellectual development of children born following a certain form of assisted reproduction is being compared with that of children conceived normally, inviting all of the children to attend on the same morning might result, for example, in the parents of controls discovering that their neighbour's child has been conceived artificially. Similarly, medical or psychological research should not normally be conducted on school premises where teachers or other pupils may become aware of facts about the participants to which they are not entitled, or start asking embarrassing questions.

Participant information sheets are another potential source of a breach of confidentiality and researchers should warn participants of the need to keep the sheets locked away out of sight of unexpected visitors.

The identity of participants must obviously never be directly revealed in any publication or presentation describing the results of the research, but care should also be taken, particularly in the reporting of genetics studies, to ensure that no information, such as a family tree, is revealed that could lead to individuals indirectly being identified. In reporting studies on very rare conditions, particular care should also be taken to avoid inadvertently identifying individuals or families. If there is any chance of a patient being identified by friends or relatives as a result of a published account, their informed consent must first be obtained (Smith 1995).

8

Clinical trials

Development of a new drug or procedure

Before it can be marketed, a new drug must be shown to be safe and effective. Clinical trials are therefore organised involving, firstly, healthy volunteers and, subsequently, patients to test the safety and usefulness of a promising new treatment or procedure. While many clinical trials are designed to evaluate new drugs, for example a new antibiotic or a new combination of drugs aimed at killing cancer cells, other trials might compare different radiation treatments or surgical procedures, for example, a comparison of radical surgery versus local excision for the treatment of breast cancer.

Multicentre drug trials are organised by pharmaceutical companies as a necessary part of gaining data on the safety and effectiveness of the drug to satisfy the licensing authorities, so that it can be licensed and marketed. Trials of drugs or procedures may also be organised by medical charities or professional organisations.

The International Conference on Harmonisation, *Guideline for Good Clinical Practice*

Good clinical practice is a standard for the design, conduct, performance, monitoring, auditing, recording, analysis and reporting of clinical trials sponsored by the pharmaceutical industry, so that there is public assurance that the data and reported results are credible and accurate, and that the rights, integrity and confiden-tiality of trial subjects are protected. Good clinical practice would be better termed good clinical *research* practice as research is what it refers to, but the expression, good clinical practice, seems to have stuck. The ethical principles enshrined in the Declaration of Helsinki (World Medical Association 1996), including the impor-tance of obtaining the patient's informed consent to experimental procedures and the prior review of research proposals by an ethics committee, have been incorporated into good clinical practice and are basic to its operation.

Drug development regulations vary in detail between nations, causing problems for pharmaceutical companies wishing to ensure that the conduct of their trials would satisfy the licensing authorities in different countries. The US Food and Drug Administration guidelines (Allen 1991) for instance require much closer reporting to the ethics committee than did the former European Community (Commission of the European Communities 1990). Differing requirements could result in experiments being repeated resulting in the unnecessary exposure of patients/volun-teers to procedures and drugs, and unnecessary use of animals. The objective of the International Conference on Harmonisation (ICH) *Guideline for Good Clinical Practice* is to provide a unified standard for the European Union, Japan and the USA to facilitate the mutual acceptance of clinical data by the regulatory authorities in these jurisdictions that comprise the world's largest pharmaceutical markets. The guideline was developed taking into account the good clinical practice guidelines of the European Union, the USA, and Japan, as well as those of Australia, Canada, the Nordic coun-tries and the World Health Organization (WHO).

The ICH guideline came into effect on 17 January 1997. A European directive has been drafted with the aim of providing in 1999, a legal framework to enable Member States to incorporate ICH good clinical practice into their own legislation.

The basic principles of the international guideline (ICH 1996) are given below. For ease of cross referencing, the numbering in brackets (e.g. DHI.4) refers to the corresponding principles of the Declaration of Helsinki (World Medical Association 1996).

●●●● The principles of the International Conference on Harmonisation *Guideline for Good Clinical Practice* (1996)

- ► Clinical trials should be conducted in accordance with the ethical principles that have their origin in the Declaration of Helsinki, and that are consistent with GCP and the applicable regulatory requirement(s).

- ► Before a trial is initiated, foreseeable risks and inconveniences should be weighed against the anticipated benefit for the individual trial subject and society. A trial should be initiated and continued only if the anticipated benefits justify the risk. (DH I.4.)

- ► The rights, safety and well-being of the trial subjects are the most important considerations and should prevail over the interests of science and society. (DH I.5.)

- ► The available non-clinical and clinical information on an investigational product should be adequate to support the proposed clinical trial. (DH I.1.)

- ► Clinical trials should be scientifically sound, and described in a clear, detailed protocol. (DH I.1.)

- ► A trial should be conducted in compliance with the protocol that has received prior institutional review board (IRB)/independent ethics committee (IEC) approval/ favourable opinion. (DH I.2.)

- ► The medical care given to, and medical decisions made on behalf of, subjects should always be the responsibility of a qualified physician or, when appropriate, of a qualified dentist. (DH I.3.)

- ► Each individual involved in conducting a trial should be qualified by education, training, and experience to perform his or her respective task(s). (DHI.3.)

- ► Freely given consent should be obtained from every subject prior to clinical trial participation. (DH I.9.)

- ► All clinical trial information should be recorded, handled and stored in a way that allows its accurate reporting, interpretation and verification. (DH I.8.)

► The confidentiality of records that could identify subjects should
  be protected, respecting the privacy and confidentiality rules in
  accordance with the applicable regulatory requirement(s). (DH I.6.)
► Investigational products should be manufactured, handled and
  stored in accordance with applicable good manufacturing practice.
  They should be used in accordance with the approved protocol.
► Systems with procedures that assure the quality of every aspect of
  the trial should be implemented.

Mutual responsibilities of investigators and ethics committees

No subject should be admitted to a trial before the institutional
review board or independent ethics committee has formally
approved it. Before initiating a trial, the investigator/institution
should have written and dated approval from the ethics committee
for the trial protocols, the written informed consent form, the
subject recruitment procedure (e.g., advertisements) and any
written information to be provided to subjects.

Responsibilities of the institutional review board/independent ethics committee

In contrast to the European good clinical practice guideline
(Commission of the European Communities 1990), in the ICH
guideline (ICH 1996) the responsibilities of the ethics committee as
they apply to clinical trials are clearly defined. The key requirements outlined in section 3.1 (ICH 1996) include:

► Safeguard the rights, safety and well-being of all trial subjects.
  Special attention should be paid to trials that may include
  vulnerable subjects, such as children and those with learning
  disabilities.
► Obtain the following documents –
  (a) the trial protocol and amendments;
  (b) written informed consent forms and consent form updates,
      that the investigator proposes to use in the trial;

 (c) subject recruitment procedures (e.g., advertisements);

 (d) written information to be provided to subjects;

 (e) the investigator's brochure and any updates;

 (f) available safety information;

 (g) information about payments provided to subjects;

 (h) information about compensation available to subjects;

 (i) the investigator's current curriculum vitae and/or other documentation evidencing qualifications;

 (j) any other documents that the ethics committee may need to fulfil its responsibilities.

► Review a proposed clinical trial within a reasonable time and document its views in writing, clearly identifying the trial, the documents reviewed and the dates of its decisions.

► Consider the qualifications of the investigator for the proposed trial, as documented by a current curriculum vitae and/or by any other relevant documentation.

► Conduct continuing review of each ongoing trial at intervals appropriate to the degree of risk to human subjects, but at least once per year.

► Request more information when the additional information would add meaningfully to the protection of the rights, safety and/or well-being of the subjects.

► When a non-therapeutic trial is to be carried out with the consent of the subject's legally acceptable representative, determine that the proposed protocol and/or other document(s) adequately address relevant ethical concerns.

► When informed consent cannot be obtained, the ethics committee should determine that the proposed protocol and/or other document(s) adequately address relevant ethical concerns.

► Review both the amount and method of payment to subjects to ensure that neither presents problems or coercion or undue influence on the trial subjects. Payments to a subject should be prorated and not wholly contingent on completion of the trial by the subject.

► Ensure that information regarding payment to subjects, including the methods, amounts and schedule of payment to trial subjects, is set forth in the written informed consent form and any other written information to be provided to subjects. The way payment will be prorated should be specified.

▶ The institutional review board/independent ethics committee should provide its written procedures and membership lists when asked to do so by investigators, sponsors or regulatory authorities.

▶ In studies involving emergency situations where prior consent is not possible the ethics committee should ensure that the relevant ethical concerns have been adequately addressed.

▶ Under ICH (s.3.4), the ethics committee should now retain all relevant records (e.g., written procedures, membership lists, list of occupations/affiliations of members, submitted documents, minutes of meetings and correspondence) for a period of at least three years after completion of the trial and make them available upon request from the regulatory authority(ies).

Responsibilities of the investigator in regard to the ethics committee

The ICH guideline (ICH 1996) emphasises the responsibility of the investigator to keep the ethics committee informed of developments in the study following approval.

▶ The investigator should submit written summaries of the trial status to the ethics committee annually, or more frequently, if requested by the ethics committee. (s.4.10.1.)

▶ No deviations from, or changes to, the protocol should be initiated without prior written ethics committee approval, except when necessary to eliminate immediate hazards to the subjects, or when the changes involve only logistical or administrative aspects of the trial (e.g., change of monitors, telephone numbers etc.). (s.4.5.2.)

▶ The investigator should report promptly to the ethics committee (s.3.3.8) –

    (a) deviations from, or changes to the protocol to eliminate immediate hazards to the trial subjects;

(b) changes increasing the risk to subjects and/or affecting significantly the conduct of the trial;

(c) all adverse drug reactions that are both serious and unexpected;

(d) new information that may affect adversely the safety of the subjects or the conduct of the trial.

The above is no more than a summary of some of the key features of the ICH *Guideline for Good Clinical Practice*. A copy of the complete document should be obtained and read by all researchers and others involved in clinical trials (see under, 'Useful Addresses').

The process of developing a new therapeutic drug

The development of a new therapeutic drug is an extremely time consuming and costly affair. It typically takes around 12 years from the synthesis of a new drug until it can be prescribed to patients. As patents normally only last for 20 years, this gives drug companies very little time in which to make a profit. Most new drugs in fact never recoup their development costs. In an effort to gain extra years before their patent expires, drug companies are making concerted efforts to reduce substantially the research and development period.

The process begins with the identification of a new substance that may have a beneficial property that would make it useful in treating certain illnesses. Reaching this stage is likely to have already taken many years of painstaking research. Having identified the drug, it then has to be obtained in sufficient amounts. This may mean extracting it from plants, animals or bacteria, or making it chemically in the laboratory from another substance that is already available. Methods then have to be devised to obtain the drug in a high state of purity.

Animal testing

Initial studies may be carried out on single cells or tissue preparations. If the results warrant further investigation, the substance may then be tested on animals to see whether it produces the desired effect, like reducing blood pressure or overcoming an infection. Sometimes the disease, or a model for it, has first to be induced in the animals.

If it still looks promising, the next stage is to test its safety by feeding it in increasing doses to animals to see whether it produces any harmful effects. It is normal practice to do these studies in two species, a rodent, typically rats, and a non-rodent, typically dogs. The animals are usually killed at the end so that their liver, kidneys and other organs can be examined in detail for signs of damage.

Animal testing obviously raises significant ethical considerations in itself. Nowadays, an increasing number of 'new' drugs are simply minor modifications to the structure of old ones designed, for instance, to enable them to be absorbed more quickly from the intestines into the blood or to slow the rate at which they are eliminated from the body. In such cases, animal testing is often of limited value. Animal testing is not legally required for all new drugs in Britain, but tight government guidelines mean that regulating bodies would be unlikely to accept a new drug without evidence of these preliminary tests. The Declaration of Helsinki (World Medical Association 1996) states that '*the welfare of animals used for research must be respected.*' Further discussion of this important aspect of medical research is, however, outside the scope of this book.

Toxicity test findings together with other animal test results are then closely examined to see whether the drug can be tested on humans. The results have to be extrapolated with care, because of the diverse ways in which each species responds to different drugs. Classical examples are penicillin which is lethal to guinea pigs; and thalidomide which produces birth defects when taken during pregnancy in women and some other species of mammal but not in others. Clinical trials only begin after preliminary studies in the laboratory and on animals have shown promising results.

The licensing authority

Before trials on patients can begin, proposals for the study must go before the national licensing authority and gain the appropriate certification. For investigators in the UK, this is the Medicines Control Agency or the European Medicines Evaluation Agency and in the USA, this is the Food and Drug Administration. All the data on the animal tests plus the details of the doctors who are conducting the trials are submitted. If the Medicines Control Agency has no objections and approval has been given by the appropriate medical research ethics committees the clinical trials can go ahead. To determine what studies require prior notification to the Medicines Control Agency and under what scheme, readers are referred to the appropriate government guidelines (Medicines Act 1968 available from the Medicines Control Agency, see under 'Useful addresses') and to the summary provided by Wiffen and Reynolds (1997). Interestingly, products comprising viable human tissue, such as cultured cells to assist wound healing, fall outside the scope of both the 1968 Medicines Act and the Medical Devices Directive (93/42/EEC) and are thus, at the time of writing, unregulated within the UK (Gentzkow et al. 1996). Nevertheless, researchers would be expected to make the appropriate organisation, such as the Medical Devices Agency, aware of the development of any such product.

The setting up of a study by a pharmaceutical company includes the following steps:

► Production of the detailed study protocol including patients or volunteer information sheets and case report forms.
► The selection of sites. This may initially involve trawling publication lists to find researchers who are experienced in this kind of study, or approaching researchers who have worked well with the company in the past.
► Submission of proposals to the appropriate ethics committee.
► Contractual arrangements with various departments within the hospital.
► Site initiation visit.

Clinical trials
These trials are usually conducted in steps or phases.

Phase I trials: testing in healthy volunteers
The first stage of a drug trial in which a new drug is administered to patients is known as a Phase I trial. Unless the drug is particularly toxic, for example a new drug for cancer chemotherapy, in these early trials it will be given to healthy volunteers rather than to patients. Doses are given in gradually increasing amounts to different volunteers. It will already be known what doses produce harmful effects in animals, and the first doses to humans are kept well below this.

In such trials, the volunteers will be kept under close observation while the drug is administered and for a period afterwards. The main aim of this stage is to ensure that the drug is safe and that there are no unacceptable side-effects. Another aim is to investigate the rate at which it is absorbed into the body (usually from the intestines into the blood) and then removed from the body. This kind of research is typically done in specialist research units located within hospitals with the facilities for constantly monitoring the heart rate, blood pressure and the general health of volunteers.

The Phase I trial tests the new drug against a placebo. As the subjects are healthy volunteers, the use of placebo at this stage raises none of the ethical issues that are discussed fully in Chapter 10. The allocation is random and 'blind', which means that participants do not know which treatment they are on. In this way, any side-effects of the new drug can be distinguished from those which, like headache, nausea or intestinal disturbances, may be due to the unaccustomed atmosphere or food of a hospital ward. These Phase I trials typically take up to two years.

Phase II trials: first administration to patients
The Phase II trials are those in which the drug is given to patients for the first time. They typically involve up to a few hundred patients and are placebo controlled.

If it has been established from the Phase I trial using healthy volunteers that the drug has no obvious risks associated with it, the aim now is to establish whether it is active against the disease, its short-term safety in patients, and the best dose to give to patients. For example, if the aim is to reduce the patient's blood pressure to within a certain range, the dose would be increased (up to a certain limit) until the appropriate reduction is brought about. If the initial small-scale studies appear promising, trials will then be conducted on larger numbers of patients. If not, it is unlikely that any more trials will take place.

Early access to a new treatment

Participants in a clinical trial are the first patients to receive a new drug when it becomes available. In some cases, the new drug may be the only one that is available for treating a disease, or it may have potential benefits over existing treatments. While it is possible that the new drug may turn out to be disappointing, the researchers usually have a good reason to believe that it will be more effective for at least some classes of patient or have fewer side-effects than the current treatments. It has to be emphasised, however, that until clinical trials are conducted, no one knows whether the new treatment being tested will prove to be better than treatments already available. There is always the chance that it will turn out to be ineffective or do more harm than good, and it certainly will not benefit patients in the placebo group.

Phase III trials: further testing on patients

From the manufacturer's point of view, the main aim of this phase is to gain enough information from enough patients over a sufficient period of time to gain a licence to sell the new drug. This phase will only be undertaken if there is sufficient evidence from the Phase II trials to suggest that the new drug is beneficial to the patients and that the risk of side-effects is acceptable.

At this stage the manufacturer hopes to be able to demonstrate that their drug has some advantage over those currently on the market, such as being more effective at treating the condition, having fewer side-effects, or available at lower cost. Phase III trials therefore almost always compare the new drug with an existing drug in an effort to demonstrate its superiority. In such trials the patients are typically split into groups. The first group receive the new drug, the second group receive a currently used drug and, if acceptable, a third group is given a placebo. To avoid bias, neither the patients nor their doctors usually know which treatment they are being given – a double-blind study – although the doctor must be able to find out quickly which group is which in an emergency.

Phase III trials require large numbers of patients, typically a thousand or more, to be studied over a long period of time and are therefore conducted in many different hospitals or family doctor practices as national or international multicentre trials. They take an average of four years.

The results of the trials are sent to the national drug licensing body of the country concerned. If the committee agrees that the new treatment is effective and safe it is licensed for marketing. For the granting of a product licence, UK companies can now apply to the European Medicines Evaluation Agency (EMEA) instead of the Medicines Control Agency. An EMEA licence is valid in all European Union member states.

Phase IV trials

These trials are conducted after a product licence has been granted and the product has been marketed, and should have at least one of the following aims:

▶ To show that the product continues to work in prolonged use.
▶ To identify any side-effects resulting from prolonged use.
▶ To establish whether it continues to have an advantage over other drugs when used in the long-term.
▶ To identify the possibility of overdose and possible misuse.

- To identify alternative doses (e.g., once daily instead of twice daily) and means of administering the drug (e.g., by mouth rather than injection).
- To establish why some patients fail to respond to the drug.

With Phase IV trials, it is important for ethics committees to ensure that the research is valid and capable of yielding useful information, and not simply marketing exercises aimed at introducing the product to as many centres as possible (La Puma et al 1995). A placebo is not usually involved in this phase. If the intention is to use a marketed drug to treat a condition for which it was not originally designed, the drug will need to undergo new Phase III trials to obtain a further licence.

Reporting of adverse events and *serious* adverse events

In a drug trial, investigators are responsible for providing the pharmaceutical company and ethics committee with information concerning any findings that suggest significant hazards, contraindications, side-effects or precautions relevant to the safety of the drug under investigation.

Definition of an adverse event

An adverse event can be defined as any:

- unintended, unfavourable clinical sign or symptom;
- clinically relevant deterioration in any laboratory assessment (e.g., haematological, biochemical, hormonal) or other clinical test (e.g., ECG, X-ray) even when symptoms are not present;
- new illness or disease or the deterioration of existing disease or illness.

These data must be recorded on the appropriate company report forms regardless of whether or not there is thought to be a reasonable possibility that the event may have been caused by the study or drug under investigation.

Definition of a serious adverse event or serious adverse drug reaction

A serious adverse event or drug reaction includes any experience or event that:

▶ Results in death.

▶ Is life-threatening – a 'life-threatening event' is present when the patient was, in the view of the investigator, at immediate risk of death from the event as it occurred. This definition does *not* include an event which hypothetically might have caused death if it were more severe.

▶ Requires the subject to be admitted to hospital or, if already in hospital, prolongs the stay. Planned admission to hospital for treatment of a pre-existing condition that did not worsen during the study is not considered an adverse event. However, complications which occur during the hospitalisation are to be regarded as adverse events and if a complication prolongs hospitalisation then the event should be recorded as a *serious* adverse event.

▶ Results in persistent or significant disability or incapacity.

▶ Is a congenital anomaly/birth defect in the offspring of a patient who received the study drug.

The above represents the ICH good clinical practice definition (ICH 1996, s.1.50). Many pharmaceutical companies also include the following:

▶ Cancer.

▶ An event resulting from an overdose of the drug – an overdose is the consumption (whether accidental or intentional) of a dose greater than the highest dose defined in the protocol which results in signs or symptoms. If no adverse signs or symptoms occur, the case is not treated as a serious adverse event.

► Pregnancy.

Unexpected adverse events

An unexpected adverse effect is any that is not identified in the investigational brochure.

Reporting of serious adverse events

To the pharmaceutical company

Life-threatening adverse events and deaths, whether or not expected or considered to be associated with the treatment, must be notified by the investigator to the pharmaceutical company within 24 hours. All data immediately available must be reported. Following initial notification the investigator must then record all additional information and fax or mail a copy of the completed adverse event reporting forms within 48 hours.

For all other serious adverse events and pregnancies, the details must be notified within 48 hours.

To the ethics committee

All serious adverse events whether occurring locally or at other sites must be reported to the institutional review board or research ethics committee, with the minimum of delay.

This chapter has focused on drug trials, but the importance of rapidly reporting serious adverse events to the ethics committee applies equally to all kinds of research. The study must immediately be suspended if there is any possibility that subjects may be harmed, until the question of whether the serious adverse event was related to the study has been resolved.

Pharmaceutical companies must report all serious adverse events to the regulatory authorities.

Post-marketing monitoring

Even after new medicines are licensed and available for routine prescription their safety must continue to be monitored. One such scheme developed in the UK is the Yellow Card system. When a patient receiving a medicine suffers an adverse reaction, their usual doctor reports this on the special postage paid form, the Yellow Card to the Committee on Safety of Medicines.

For newer drugs, doctors are asked to report any adverse or unexpected event, however minor, which could conceivably be attributed to the drug. Reports should be made even if the doctor is uncertain whether or not it was the drug to blame.

For established drugs, doctors are asked *not* to report well known, relatively minor side-effects such as dry mouth, constipation or nausea, but to restrict their reporting to any suspected adverse drug reaction that was potentially damaging, incapacitating or lethal. These must always be reported even if it is well documented that the drug can occasionally have these effects.

Whenever an infant is born with a congenital abnormality or when there is a malformed aborted fetus, doctors must report all drugs (including those bought over the counter by the patient) taken by the mother during pregnancy.

As the doctor is prescribing the drug because it is thought to be the best treatment for the patients, post-market monitoring is defined as standard clinical care rather than research and can be done without the patient's informed consent, even if it involves extracting information from their case records. Strict rules of confidentiality will obviously still apply.

Pharmaceutical companies may also conduct more formal assessments of the clinical safety of marketed medicines, known as SAMM (Safety Assessment of Marketed Medicines) (Association of the British Pharmaceutical Industry 1988, 1993).

9

Research with healthy volunteers

The golden rule is that healthy volunteers must never be exposed to more than minimal risk, i.e. the risks of a typical persons'daily life.

Justification for research with volunteers

Many basic biochemical, physiological and psychological studies are carried out with healthy volunteers rather than patients. When such studies have no immediate prospect of yielding anything of therapeutic benefit it is generally more acceptable to use healthy volunteers than to trouble sick people.

Some kinds of study, by their very nature, can only be done on healthy volunteers. A new vaccine, for instance, will have to be tested on healthy members of the population to see if it prevents them from contracting the infection that it is designed to protect against.

As explained in the previous chapter, Phase I volunteer trials usually constitute the first stage in the process of testing a new drug on humans. Many drugs fail to meet the basic criteria, for example, for not effectively being absorbed from the gut into the blood stream, at the volunteer phase and are never tried out on patients. Performing the preliminary tests on healthy volunteers therefore avoids raising false hopes in patients, or giving them an ineffective treatment when something better is already available. Another common problem avoided, if it did turn out to be effective, is the likelihood that it will no longer be available at the end of the trial owing to its limited availability, cost or because it has not yet satisfied the licensing regulations.

It is also easier in healthy volunteers to identify the side-effects of the medicine being tested, whereas in patients it may be difficult to distinguish side-effects from symptoms of the illness. Moreover, placebos can be used at will in healthy volunteers without raising the ethical issues associated with their use in patients. The early stage in the development of a new medicine also involves constant monitoring and frequent blood sampling, an additional burden that it might be unfair to inflict on patients in poor health.

At the other extreme, some medicines can never be tried out on volunteers to assess their safety, because it is already known that they have significant side-effects or a high risk of provoking serious adverse events. New treatments for cancer, which may result in increased susceptibility to infection or increased hair loss, fall into this category. Only patients already at risk of experiencing these side-effects from the standard treatment could be expected to consider participating.

Recruitment of volunteers

Volunteers should always be recruited of their own free will. Potential participants should be made aware of the possibility of volunteering by a general notice, rather than by being approached directly, so that the initiative for volunteering rests entirely with the individual. This is particularly important in the case of junior members of staff and students. They must never be made to volunteer against their wishes out of fear that their career prospects or examination marks might be adversely affected if they fail to come forward.

Financial inducements must be avoided

As stated in the World Health Organization (WHO) guidelines, payments to participants should not be so large as to induce prospective subjects to participate against their better judgement (CIOMS/WHO 1993, g.4).

As volunteers must never be exposed to more than minimal risk, payments for undergoing risk would be inappropriate and should never be made. If remuneration is available, it should not be mentioned in recruiting advertisements, although it is acceptable to mention that travelling expenses and other out-of-pocket expenses will be met. Where a payment for inconvenience is made in addition to out-of-pocket expenses, in order to avoid creating a significant financial inducement, this should not exceed the average income for the area.

In reality, for many healthy volunteers, money is bound to be an added inducement. Healthy volunteers tend to be students and other less well off members of society who are likely to see participation in a drug trial as a means of funding an annual holiday or paying off some of their debts. Despite this, we should not underestimate the amount of altruism involved. In the UK, where medical care is available to all regardless of income, low-income volunteers are as likely as anyone else to benefit in the future from any new treatments arising from the research. In areas of the world where the availability of medical care depends on income, the situation is different. The question must then be asked whether it conforms to our concept of justice to employ mainly disadvantaged subjects to test a new drug that their poverty would deny them access to should it prove of benefit and be needed by them (Belmont 1979; CIOMS/WHO 1993, g.10).

Susceptible groups of healthy volunteers

Child volunteers
There is universal agreement that research should not be done on children if comparable research can be done on adults (Department of Health 1991, s.4.1; British Paediatric Association 1992, p.3; CIOMS/WHO 1993, g.5; Royal College of Physicians 1996, s.8.5).

This does not entirely exclude research on healthy child volunteers. It might be justified in non-invasive studies where the potential benefit is to children rather than adults. A new method of monitoring infants at risk of cot death would have to be tried out in healthy, low risk 'volunteers' first, while vaccines against childhood illnesses are another obvious example. For a fuller discussion of the ethical issues surrounding research with children see Chapter 12.

Pharmacological studies of the type we have been discussing are not normally acceptable on healthy child volunteers unless the drug has previously been shown to have an acceptable safety profile in adults and there would have to be a very strong reason to justify their inclusion in such studies (Royal College of Physicians 1986a, p.7).

Volunteers with learning disability

The same basic principle applies to research with people with learning disabilities as to research with children. Research should not be done with otherwise healthy people with learning disability if it could just as well be done with those who do not have this condition (Royal College of Physicians 1986a, p.7, 1996, s.8.9; CIOMS/WHO 1993, g.6). Their inclusion as healthy volunteers in drug trials would not therefore be acceptable.

Students and junior staff

When students are recruited for studies other than those that are purely educational, the permission of the Head of the Faculty must be obtained first, and the study must be approved by a medical research ethics committee in the normal way.

Educational studies should never involve more than minimal risk, or procedures more invasive than the sampling of small amounts of blood from a vein. A typical study might involve the consumption of a modest amount of an alcoholic beverage to explore the rate at which alcohol enters and leaves the blood, dependent on the effect of food, gender, etc. While most such studies do not currently come before ethics committees in the UK, it could be argued that they should be subject to formal review, with approval for a particular class project having to be renewed, for example, every five years. Class projects should include a mechanism for ensuring that students are not forced into participating in projects which they may find distressing or which may reveal confidential information about themselves. A student with a severe skin condition for instance may not wish to expose the affected area.

Junior colleagues are also in a very vulnerable position and may fear that their career prospects will be adversely affected if they fail to volunteer for departmental projects. The ethics committees should insist that departmental volunteers are obtained by means of a general advertisement rather than being approached directly.

Prisoners as volunteers

The WHO expresses grave doubts about the wisdom of including prisoners as healthy volunteers in medical research (CIOMS/WHO 1993, g.7).

Prisoners in the UK, in contrast to some other countries, are rarely invited to participate in research as healthy volunteers. Their inclusion in drug development studies is not considered acceptable owing to the problem of obtaining freely given informed consent (Royal College of Physicians 1996, s.1.19). While it might be considered wrong to deny prisoners the right to take part in medical research of potential benefit to the whole community if they should wish, it is not usually practical to involve them, especially when the volunteer has to make several visits to the research department! A more serious ethical consideration is the difficulty of avoiding coercion by inadvertently raising the hope that participation might improve their chances of early release.

The danger also exists of raising fears in the minds of concerned citizens that prisoners are being unfairly exploited, and used for experiments that no one else would volunteer for. It is hard to imagine anyone volunteering to have cancer cells injected under the skin of their forearm to see if they developed into tumours, but this is exactly what a group of maximum security prisoners in Ohio, USA did during the 1950s, when the Henrietta Lacks (HeLa) cancer cell line was imagined to hold the key to combating cancer. 'My grandmother, my father both died of cancer. I believe the wrongs that I have done in the eyes of society might, this might make a right on it; I don't know,' and ' I done a girl a great injustice, I want to pay back a little bit' were reasons given by two of the volunteers during a filmed interview at the time. Some developed small tumours but fortunately for them none apparently developed into metastatic cancer. The results were inconclusive. It is difficult to imagine an ethics committee condoning such research today. Indeed, current US regulations require that 'the risks involved in the research are commensurate with risks that would be accepted by nonprisoner volunteers' (45 CFR, 46.305a3).

On the other hand, research with healthy prisoners may be acceptable if it is designed to be of direct benefit to them as a group, such as a comparison of the mental health of prisoners kept under different regimes, ways of maintaining their physical fitness, or research into conditions particularly affecting prisoners, for example hepatitis, alcoholism and drug addiction (45 CFR, 46.306). Participation in studies of this kind is less likely to raise hopes of early release.

Elderly volunteers

The metabolism and side-effects of a new drug may be different in elderly persons and to test it only in young volunteers may provide misleading information about the behaviour of a drug that will be used mainly in the elderly. The increased difficulty of establishing the health of the elderly means that if elderly persons are selected as healthy volunteers in drug trials, the system of monitoring needed to ensure that the drug does not harm them may need to be even more stringent than with younger volunteers. Otherwise the ethical issues surrounding the use of elderly volunteers are essentially similar to those of volunteers in general.

Ensuring that healthy volunteers really are healthy

It is the responsibility of the researcher to establish the health of the 'healthy volunteer'. Volunteers need not be in 'perfect health'. Indeed some 'healthy volunteers' are patients in hospital for a reason unrelated to the condition being studied. It is essential, however, that the study in which they are being invited to participate should not be capable of adversely affecting any condition they may have.

In pharmacological studies, the volunteers' family doctor should be approached, with the volunteers' permission, concerning their suitability to participate. If the volunteer does not agree to this, they should not be recruited.

Subjects should be screened in accordance with established professional guidelines. The Association of the British Pharmaceutical Industry guidelines, for example, state that screening should be done by a clinician who should take an appropriate medical history, including reference to allergies, smoking, alcohol or consumption of other medically active substances. The screening must take place shortly before the study begins. The medical examination should be appropriate to the study proposed including relevant blood, urine or other tests. If the history, examination or tests show any abnormality that could be associated with an increased risk for individuals if they participated in the study, the volunteer should not take part. Any evidence of drug abuse, including alcohol should also preclude acceptance of the volunteer into the study (Association of the British Pharmaceutical Industry 1990b).

Out of concern for the safety of staff and other participants in studies that involve a lot of blood handling, blood may be screened for hepatitis and HIV. In view of the profound implications of a positive result, the volunteer should give permission to this prior to the examination. A system of counselling should be in operation should any subject test positive for HIV.

Interval between studies

Measures are needed to avoid creating the professional volunteer. For example, in invasive studies there should normally be at least a three month gap between a volunteer completing participation in one study and starting another. See Chapter 6 for a fuller discussion.

Avoiding excessive collection of blood

Participation in medical research often involves donating multiple blood samples. The volume taken in a year should be limited to no more than 1.5 litres in men and 1.0 litre in women (Royal College of Physicians 1986a, p.6). Care should be taken to avoid recruiting volunteers to a study involving the removal of large amounts of blood if they have recently donated blood. Similarly, volunteers from whom a significant amount of blood has been taken during a study should be warned against donating blood for an appropriate period, typically three months, after the end of the study, and not to participate in another study for three months after that.

Insurance and compensation

Some insurance companies consider participation in medical studies to be a 'material fact' which should be mentioned in any proposal for health-related insurance. Although few volunteers are likely to take out insurance purely in anticipation of participating in research, they should be advised to check that participation does not affect any existing policies they may hold.

The investigator must provide volunteers with details of the arrangements for compensation in the unlikely event of any deterioration in their health as a result of participation in the study.

Obtain informed consent

In common with other participants, healthy volunteers must be given a volunteer information sheet clearly explaining the background to the study, what is involved for them personally and the risks involved. Healthy volunteers normally have the advantage of plenty of time in which to make up their minds and less anxiety than patients to cloud their comprehension, so a more detailed information sheet may be in order. Only after freely informed consent has been obtained from the volunteer can they be recruited into the study.

Information sheets for controls must be clearly labelled 'healthy controls'

It would be very easy for an elderly patient on being given an information sheet headed 'Biochemical Changes in Alzheimer's Disease' to imagine that he or she had been diagnosed with this condition, even though the patient was in hospital for a hip replacement and in reality was being recruited as a healthy control.

An information sheet designed for patients should not be adapted for use by controls by deleting the words referring to patients as this can lead to confusion. Great care must always be taken to ensure that healthy volunteers are in no doubt that they are being recruited as controls. They must not be allowed to imagine, even for a moment, that they are suffering from a serious condition of which they were previously unaware. To reduce this risk, investigators should always compose a distinct information sheet for controls which is clearly labelled 'Healthy Controls', or 'Healthy Volunteers'. It should also emphasise at least once in the text that they are being selected as healthy controls.

As well as misleading the participants, without these precautions, an acquaintance catching sight of an information sheet might wrongly conclude, as in the above example, that the participant has Alzheimer's disease with potentially serious consequences if the rumour got around. An unambiguous title is therefore essential.

Safety after the study

As healthy volunteers are likely to be resuming their normal lifestyle shortly after the study, they must be warned not to immediately undertake any activities which might be rendered dangerous as a result of potential side-effects of the study, such as driving or operating other dangerous machinery.

10

Are placebos ethical?

The placebo effect

A well-known difficulty with attempts to assess the value of a new treatment is that many patients who try something new tend to feel that their condition has improved, at least in the short-term, whether the treatment is actually of any benefit to them or not. This phenomenon has been studied in the past by 'treating' patients, without telling them, with inactive substances, such as capsules of sugar, and is known as the placebo effect. (Whether it was ethical to do this is another matter!)

As a result of the placebo effect, a group of patients who have been taking for example a new painkiller will probably report that they feel less pain than a comparable group who have received nothing, even if the painkiller is totally ineffective. This bias can be overcome by giving the untreated group a placebo which looks and tastes like the real thing and ensuring that neither they nor their doctor know which they are receiving, an arrangement referred to as a double-blind, placebo controlled trial.

Alternatively, patients may act as their own controls, receiving active treatment during one period and placebo during another, in what is known as a 'cross-over' design. In, for example, a project to determine the effect of an inhaled steroid treatment for asthma on the production of cortisol by the adrenal gland, patients may be asked to inhale the steroid for several days, then to inhale a placebo for a few days, and finally to inhale the steroid again. In this way it can be determined whether the level of cortisol in the blood is different while the treatment is being inhaled compared with when it is not.

Informed consent must be obtained for the use of placebo

It is essential to ensure that patients fully understand before agreeing to participate in a placebo-controlled trial that they may receive placebo instead of active treatment, either throughout the study or at some stage of it. It would be unethical to give patients the impression that they will be receiving active treatment throughout the study if this is not the case. The chance of receiving placebo must be clearly specified in the patient information sheet. Patients need not be told at exactly what stage they will receive the placebo, if revealing this would invalidate the study.

Is a placebo control always necessary?

If the response to treatment can be accurately measured by the researcher, and, unlike pain, cannot be affected by a person's mental attitude, it may be scientifically sound to compare a treated group of patients with an untreated without using a placebo. Indeed, in some cases a placebo design may not be appropriate because of the difficulty of producing a placebo indistinguishable from the treatment. The effects of the treatment, for example with a new diuretic, may also make it obvious to patients which group they are in. The study design must be made clear to prospective participants at the outset so that they are fully aware that they may be allocated to a group not receiving treatment.

An alternative to placebo: comparing a new treatment with the best available standard treatment

As far as the typical doctors seeking the best treatment for their patients are concerned, they are not usually particularly interested in whether the new drug that the company is trying to sell them is better than a placebo, in other words, better than nothing at all. What they will want to know is whether the new drug is in some way superior to that which they currently prescribe (Aspinal and Goodman, 1995). It should be more effective at treating the illness, have fewer side-effects or be easier for patients to take. But has the standard treatment ever been tested against placebo?

On the other hand, there is little point in knowing that a new drug is as good as the standard treatment, and has fewer side-effects, if it is not known whether either drug is any better than nothing at all. This raises the vexed question of whether the standard drug has ever been adequately tested against a placebo. In the past, many drugs crept into common usage without the stringent testing and large scale clinical trials that today are required before a new drug can be licensed for use. There are thus drugs of unproven efficacy and safety remaining on the market, including some heroic treatments for cancer with major side-effects.

Today, the licensing authorities such as the UK Medicines Control Agency and the US Food and Drugs Administration usually require a new drug to be compared with a placebo before they will issue a licence for it to be marketed. This applies particularly to drugs for the treatment of conditions, as for example depression, where a high proportion of cases are expected to resolve spontaneously without treatment during the period of the trial. It also applies to 'placebo-effect conditions', such as mild depression where giving an inactive substance can itself bring about improvement, perhaps as a result of the expectation of improvement and the feeling that help is at hand (Brown 1994).

In an effort to satisfy both requirements at the same time, the manufacturer may design a clinical trial to compare the new drug both with placebo *and* with a standard treatment.

Is the use of a placebo ethical?

The Declaration of Helsinki (World Medical Association 1996) states:

In any medical study, every patient – including those of a control group if any – should be assured of the best proven diagnostic and therapeutic method. This does not exclude the use of inert placebo in studies where no proven diagnostic or therapeutic method exists Article II. 3

(This reference to placebo first appeared in the 1996 amendment to the Declaration.)

The Royal College of Physicians (1990b, s.9.5) also takes the cautious view that: 'The use of a placebo or dummy treatment poses ethical problems but is often preferable to the continued use of treatments of unproven efficacy or safety'.

But what if alternatives of proven efficacy are indeed available? While the Declaration of Helsinki does not appear to allow the use of placebo in such trials, the licensing authorities, as has already been noted, usually require a new drug to be tested against placebo before they will issue a licence for it. As a result, this is the one part of the Declaration to which research ethics committees cannot always insist on strict adherence. The US Food and Drug Administration and other drug licensing authorities should look hard at their requirements for placebo arms in drugs trials where an established treatment is already available.

A placebo-controlled drug trial poses two contrasting safety issues. Firstly, the familiar one of how likely is it that patients receiving the new drug will be harmed by it and secondly, how likely is it that those on placebo will be harmed by *not* receiving any treatment? While a placebo-controlled study is acceptable and necessary when there is no satisfactory existing treatment for the illness under investigation and the benefits of the new treatment are uncertain, this situation is fairly uncommon. Some form of standard treatment is available for most common illnesses, even if it may not always be particularly effective. Consequently, in a placebo-controlled trial it will often be necessary to deprive patients in the placebo group of available treatment, either by *not* putting newly diagnosed patients on the standard treatment or by withdrawing long established patients from it. Whether this can be considered ethical will depend on the likelihood of patients being harmed by withdrawing them from the standard treatment, and how serious this harm might be.

Minor illnesses

Not all illness is life threatening and in many studies patients on placebo may 'only' have to put up with temporary pain or discomfort. For example, in a trial of a new drug for migraine, this may mean having to suffer a headache for a few hours, for Raynaud's disease, pain in the fingers, or for dyspepsia, stomach pains. When there is no risk of long-term harm, the use of placebo may be acceptable so long as participants are fully aware that they may be allocated to a group who will not receive any medication for their condition, and of the discomfort they may suffer as a result.

Participants must be clearly informed what rescue medication is available and have rapid 24-hour access to medical advice should their symptoms become unacceptable.

Serious conditions

In the development of a new treatment for a potentially serious condition where current treatments are known to be effective, it will not be so easy to justify the use of placebo. If depriving patients of effective treatment could allow the condition to get worse with serious consequences, it may be impossible to justify. Antibiotic treatment typically falls into this high-risk category. The effectiveness of a new antibiotic must therefore normally be compared with one of the many antibiotics already on the market rather than with placebo. For a similar reason, placebos cannot usually be used instead of standard chemotherapy in cancer patients. Another clear cut example is the development of a new drug to prevent the rejection of transplants which would obviously have to be compared with a standard immunosuppressant drug such as cyclosporin, as to compare it with placebo would result in rejection of the transplants in the placebo group.

More difficult ethical questions arise with conditions such as hypertension where there may be disagreement as to whether patients are likely to be harmed by the withdrawal of their current treatment. The use of placebo can also cause concern in studies of depression and other serious forms of mental illness where withdrawal of treatment could increase the risk of self-harm. As a general rule, patients should not be withdrawn from a treatment that appears to be stabilising their condition, unless they themselves wish to change due to unacceptable side-effects, inconvenience or justifiable dissatisfaction with the current treatment. An ethics committee will be unhappy with the idea that patients could be taken off satisfactory medication, which was achieving its aim without side-effects, purely for recruitment into a clinical trial of a new drug.

In those exceptional cases where researchers can justify withdrawal of treatment to their patients, to the ethics committee and to themselves, frequent monitoring of patients is essential to ensure that those on placebo do not suffer unacceptable illness or discomfort as a result of the withdrawal. When, for instance, the patient's current antihypertensive is withdrawn in order to test a new one, frequent checks are essential to ensure that the patient's blood pressure, especially that of those on placebo, does not rise above the predetermined safety limit.

The best of both worlds – placebo plus active treatment

Receipt of a placebo does not necessarily mean that the patient is being deprived of active treatment. Where the new drug tackles the disease by a different mechanism from the standard treatment, the drug or placebo can be given in addition to it. Following certain kinds of strokes, for instance, the standard treatment is to give aspirin or heparin to reduce the tendency of the blood to clot. Consider a new class of drug designed to limit the spread of damage in the brain resulting from the initial stroke. As it works by a completely different mechanism, all stroke patients can continue to receive aspirin or heparin whether they are on the new drug or placebo. Similarly, in a condition such as epilepsy where not to take any drug at all might be dangerous, a new drug would typically be given in addition to the standard treatment, not instead of it. If the new drug further reduced the number of seizures, it might then be possible to gradually withdraw the original medication.

In a study to compare two active treatments, a placebo may be used simply to disguise which treatment is being taken. In a comparison of two treatments for asthma, one inhaled and the other taken orally, it would be obvious to all concerned which was which. To avoid this, one group of patients would be given an active inhaler together with the dummy tablet, while the other group would be given a dummy inhaler and the active tablet. As no one is denied treatment, the use of placebo in such cases does not raise the usual ethical issues.

Neither are ethical issues raised by the use of placebo in basic studies involving healthy volunteers who do not require any treatment.

Is a control group always necessary?

While, in order to compare the effectiveness of a particular treatment, it is standard practice to compare patients receiving the treatment with those who are not, or with those receiving alternative treatment, there are exceptions to every rule.

For example, take the case of children with intractable speech disorders who have been seeing a speech therapist for years but who seem to have reached a plateau. A new aid has been devised to help their speech. As the children all have intractable problems and are already receiving intensive therapy, it is reasonable to assume that any progress made during the first two or three weeks of the study is due to the new equipment. Is there any need, therefore, to deprive half of the children of the opportunity to try out the new aid by keeping them as controls?

Effective controls may be impossible to obtain

In some cases, it may be virtually impossible to obtain effective controls. Taking another example from speech therapy, this time a study based on the possibility that some children with severe verbal communication difficulties may be able to communicate more effectively by the written word on a computer. The disabilities experienced by children chosen for the study are likely to have different diagnoses, the only common factor being their inability to communicate verbally. This, together with individual rates of learning, implies that the study group will not be homogenous. It is thus virtually impossible to set up an effective control group.

While purists will reject outright the idea that any study could be scientifically valid in the absence of a placebo or other control group, or indeed that such a study could even constitute research, it has to be acknowledged that much valuable information has been obtained from observational studies conducted without controls. Where there is a special problem with incorporating a control arm into the design of the study, this should be explained to the ethics committee who must then consider each case on its merits.

Invasive placebos

Examples of invasive placebos include multiple injections of inactive fluid, or the creation of a small incision in the abdomen to conceal from patients whether they had received an experimental minor operation (such as nerve ablation aimed at reducing pain) or been allocated to a control group. Such studies will need to come under the closest scrutiny by the ethics committee to determine if they are ethically acceptable. In the latter example, the risk and discomfort involved and the extent of the scarring (which might in effect be minimal with modern surgical techniques) would have to be balanced against the potential benefits.

Guidelines for the use of placebos in clinical trials

Reference to placebos in the international guidelines (International Conference on Harmonisation 1996) is surprisingly limited, while the latest Royal College of Physicians guidelines (RCP 1996, s.6.28–6.30) make only general mention. In the absence of detailed professional guidelines on the use of placebos, the following list of recommendations is offered.

▶ The use of placebo is not acceptable if patients are placed at risk of a serious deterioration in their condition as a result.

▶ It is not acceptable to withdraw patients from standard treatment, which is satisfactorily stabilising their condition, in order to place them in a study where they may receive placebo.

▶ Researchers must be able to justify the failure to implement, or to withdraw, standard treatment in order to put patients on placebo. (If it does not contain the necessary expertise amongst its members, the ethics committee must obtain an expert opinion as to whether withdrawing effective treatment is acceptable.)

▶ Relief medication, if it exists, must always be available if required, even if it means that a patient feeling the need to take it has consequently to be withdrawn from the trial.

▶ If no satisfactory relief medication exists, patients must be withdrawn from the trial if pain or other symptoms become unacceptable.

▶ Patients must be given a 24-hour phone number to ring should they feel concerned about their condition.

▶ Patients on placebo must be monitored frequently to detect at an early stage any worsening of their condition.

▶ Should a patient's condition worsen, it must be possible to quickly break the code, so that if the patient is found to be on placebo, active treatment can be initiated.

▶ Potential participants in a no-treatment or placebo-controlled trial must be fully informed that they may:
   (a) be allocated to a group that will not receive any medication for their condition;

      (b) or act as their own controls with a period spent on placebo, as well as a period spent receiving treatment;

      (c) and/or undergo a wash-out period on placebo before starting active treatment.

▶ The chance of receiving placebo must be specified.

▶ If patients are receiving standard treatment that needs to be stopped for the purpose of the study (or the initiation of standard treatment is delayed), and this is likely to result in any additional illness or discomfort, the patient information sheet must clearly state the length of time for which the standard treatment will be withdrawn (or delayed) and the possible side-effects.

▶ The use of placebo may not be acceptable in some extremely vulnerable groups, such as terminally ill cancer patients.

▶ To ensure that the placebo design is scientifically valid, the placebo must be sufficiently close in shape, size, weight, surface and internal colour, texture, taste and smell to the active preparation for the difference not to be detectable by patients and researchers.

▶ Invasive placebos, such as injections of inactive substances, must involve no more than minimal risk, and their nature be clearly explained to the participants.

11

Arrangements for compensation

What happens in the rare event of something going wrong in a clinical trial? In the event of death, injury or lasting disability occurring as a result of participation, who will accept responsibility for compensation? A medical research ethics committee should only approve a project if it is satisfied that the arrangements for compensation are satisfactory. Patients and volunteers for their part are advised only to participate in a study that may carry an element of risk if they have been clearly informed of the arrangements for compensation and are satisfied with them.

Clinical trials sponsored by a pharmaceutical company

The requirements in each country will differ and, apart from pointing this out, the International Conference on Harmonisation (ICH) *Guideline for Good Clinical Practice* fails to deal with the issue of compensation (ICH, 1996 s.5.8).

In the UK, it is generally accepted that arrangements for compensation in the event of injury occurring in a trial sponsored by a pharmaceutical company whether by negligence or not, *must* as a minimum, comply with the guidelines of the Association of British Pharmaceutical Industry (ABPI 1991).

The ABPI guidelines state that compensation should be paid when, on the balance of probabilities, the injury can be attributed either to the administration of a medicinal product under trial or to any clinical intervention or procedure, such as the taking of blood or tissue samples, which would not have occurred but for the inclusion of the patient in the trial. Compensation should also be paid where the injury is not directly due to the medicine but to any procedures that have been carried out in an effort to treat adverse reactions to the medicine. It should also be paid to children injured in utero through the participation of their mother.

Under the ABPI guidelines, compensation should be paid without patients needing to prove that the company or the investigator was negligent and regardless of whether or not they were informed that there was a slight risk of such injury occurring as a result of participation, and consented nevertheless. This is referred to as a 'no fault' claim.

It should be understood that the ABPI guidelines were designed to apply only to research on unlicensed products, not to research on products once they have received their product license, nor to trials that have not been initiated or sponsored directly by the company concerned. Neither do they apply to Phase I trials on healthy volunteers. In such trials alternative arrangements must be in place.

Limitations to the compensation

Under the ABPI guidelines, there are important limitations to the compensation. Minor injury, temporary pain or discomfort, or minor or curable complaints, do not qualify for compensation. No compensation will be paid if: (a) a medicine or product fails to have its intended affect; (b) the condition, during the trial of a patient receiving placebo worsens; (c) the injury has arisen due to the doctor not conforming to the requirements of the company protocol; (d) the doctor fails to deal adequately with an adverse reaction to the drug; or (e) the injury has arisen through contributory negligence by the patient due, for instance, to exceeding the stated dose.

In assessing the amount of compensation, various factors will be taken into account, including the severity and persistence of the injury. It should in general terms be consistent with the level of damages commonly awarded for similar injuries by an English court in cases where legal liability is admitted. Compensation may be considerably reduced where the patient is suffering from a life threatening illness for which established treatments carry a serious risk of adverse reactions and where the new treatment would be expected to carry similar risks of which the patient was made fully aware.

A full copy of the current guidelines can be obtained from the ABPI (see under 'Some Useful addresses'). The researcher should make copies of the ABPI guidelines available to patients on request.

In view of the limitations, it is essential that the researcher and employing institutions have adequate insurance to cover claims arising from, for example, negligence or non-compliance with the protocol.

In the UK, all trials sponsored by pharmaceutical companies must comply *fully* with the ABPI guidelines. The ethics committee must scrutinise the company's indemnity arrangements carefully to ensure that no attempts further to limit liability have crept in, such as a putting the onus on the patient to reveal past illnesses or drug reactions that could affect their response to the treatment under test. Neither should any attempt be made to limit compensation to the cost of treating the injury (which in the UK is free to all patients) resulting from participation in the trial.

The importance of ensuring that sponsors do not attempt to limit their legal liability in this way in the USA is emphasised by the Department of Health and Human Services regulations which state that: 'No informed consent, whether oral or written, may include any exculpatory language through which the subject or the representative is made to waive or appear to waive any of the subject's legal rights, or releases or appears to release the researcher, the sponsor, the institution or its agents from liability for negligence' (45 CFR, 46.116; 21 CFR, 50.20).

Studies *not* sponsored by a pharmaceutical company

When research is initiated not by a pharmaceutical company but by another institutional sponsor or an individual researcher, it is their duty to ensure that their insurance arrangements are adequate to compensate patients or volunteers injured physically or emotionally as a result of participation in their study.

Where the researcher holds a contract with, as for example in the UK, the health authority, National Health Service Trust, hospital, or other institution and is undertaking research in terms of this contract, the research must be approved by the management of the institution. Such approval should constitute acceptance of liability for negligence and *must* be obtained before research commences.

No fault insurance

It should be emphasised that insurance cover for negligence alone is far from being sufficient protection for the participant. Researchers should ensure that the terms of their insurance cover do not contain any limitations beyond those set out in the ABPI guidelines. Although they were designed specifically for Phase II and Phase III pharmaceutical trials, similar guidelines should, as far as possible, be adopted whether the study is sponsored by a pharmaceutical company or is home grown, and regardless of what type of study it is. In particular, compensation must always be available when, on the balance of probabilities, the injury was due to participation in a research study, whether or not any negligence was involved.

Patients and volunteers should not have to *sue* in order to get compensation in the event of injury occurring during a study. Researchers, their sponsors and employers owe it to those who kindly agree to participate in their research to have insurance cover that enables them to be compensated without having to risk their life savings and mental health in an effort to prove negligence through the courts. Such cover should allow compensation to be awarded whether the injury is due to the negligence of the researcher, or just bad luck (and preferably without delaying tactics by all concerned to avoid paying it). On the rare occasions where such arrangements do not exist, patients must be clearly informed of the fact before they agree to participate.

While insurance arrangements for research in Britain must conform to the guidelines of the ABPI, these must be taken as representing only the minimum protection for patients. Individual companies and organisations in the UK and in other countries may have compensation guidelines that exceed the requirements of the ABPI to the greater benefit of patients. These may then set a standard for all studies in those countries and elsewhere.

12

Research with children, seriously ill patients, persons with learning disability and other vulnerable groups

Article I.11 of the Declaration of Helsinki (World Medical Association 1996) states:

> In the case of legal incompetence, informed consent should be obtained from the legal guardian in accordance with national legislation. Where physical or mental incapacity makes it impossible to obtain informed consent, or where the subject is a minor, permission from the responsible relative replaces that of the subject in accordance with national legislation. Whenever the minor child is in fact able to give informed consent, the minor's consent must be obtained in addition to the consent of the minor's legal guardian.

Not everyone is capable of giving informed consent. These special groups include: babies, infants and younger children; older children with only partial ability to appreciate what they are being asked to do; people with learning disability; people with severe psychiatric illness; people who are seriously ill, with severe pain or distress; people who are terminally ill; the frail elderly; people who are unconscious or comatose; and anyone else whose circumstances make them especially vulnerable.

Only when research definitely cannot be carried out with anyone else should researchers invite or allow those who are unable to give consent to participate. Thus, if an investigator is conducting research on asthma and the tenth patient presenting at the clinic happens to belong to a group unable to give informed consent, no attempt should be made to recruit that patient. In some cases, however, there may be no alternative. In order to evaluate the benefits of a new drug for the treatment of Alzheimer's disease, once the initial safety and pharmacological testing on healthy volunteers have been done, it will have to be given to patients with this condition. Similarly, methods to improve the survival of premature infants can only be applied to this age group.

Each of these vulnerable groups will in turn be discussed fully in an effort to identify the key ethical issues raised by research involving them. This chapter should be read in conjunction with Chapter 4.

Children

Research should never be carried out *on* children, but *with* them

The World Health Organization (WHO) takes the view that: 'The participation of children is indispensable for research into diseases of childhood and conditions to which children are particularly susceptible' (CIOMS/WHO 1993, g.5). The British Paediatric Association (BPA 1992, p.3)agrees that: 'Research involving children is important for the benefit of all children and should be supported, encouraged and constituted in an ethical manner'. The US Department of Health and Human Services also supports ethical research with children. (45 CFR, 46.401–46.409). It warns, however, that: 'Research should only be done on children if comparable research on adults could not answer the same question'. The WHO (CIOMS/WHO 1993, g.5), Royal College of Physicians (RCP 1996, s.8.5) and the Department of Health (DoH 1991, s.4.1) share this view.

In order to obtain ethical approval for research with children, an investigator will therefore need to provide adequate justification for carrying out the study with children rather than adults. A major justification for research with children arises from the fact that children should not be given medicines that have not been adequately evaluated in the age group concerned (Committee for

Proprietary Medicinal Products (CPMP) 1997 s.1.1). It has to be established that a treatment beneficial in adults is not harmful to children who may be more susceptible to the side-effects of certain medicines at sensitive stages of growth and development. Steroid treatments marketed for use in adults with asthma, for instance, could not automatically be prescribed to children who, during critical stages of hormonally-regulated development are more susceptible to their side-effects. Similarly, anticonvulsant therapy may have harmful effects if given during early development of the central nervous system.

Research with children is also essential to establish the correct dose of medicines already used in adults. Simply adjusting for size is rarely adequate as children differ from adults in the rate at which they metabolise and eliminate some medicines – young infants may eliminate medicines more slowly due to immaturity of their liver and renal systems while older infants and children eliminate some medicines more quickly.

Clinical trials have therefore to be conducted to assess the safety and correct doses of medicines to be used in children, but only after trials have indicated an acceptable safety profile in adults. In the case of childhood conditions such as neonatal apnoea, growth hormone deficiency, paediatric tumours, the development of vaccines against childhood infections or the development of infant feeds, research can only be done on children. Even with childhood illnesses, the preliminary safety testing of new drugs should, whenever feasible, be done on adults. In general, safety studies should be conducted first in animals, then in adults and subsequently in children (CPMP 1997, s.1.3a), beginning with older children before extending the trial to younger children and then to infants.

Must research with children be aimed at benefiting the participants?

In the case of a clinical trial of a new drug, a child should normally stand to gain some benefit (CPMP 1997 s.1.1), in accord with the Declaration of Helsinki principle that concern for the interests of the individual must always prevail over those of science and society.

A research procedure which is not intended directly to benefit the child participant is not necessarily unethical, however, so long as it is designed to throw light on childhood illnesses, which may benefit children in the future, and so long as it carries no more than minimal risk (BPA 1992, p.3-4; CIOMS/WHO 1993, g.5; RCP 1996, s.8.7). The US Department of Health and Human Services goes a little further and will conduct or fund research 'where the risk represents *a minor* increase over minimal risk' (author's emphasis) so long as the research is aimed at obtaining a greater understanding of the subjects' condition (45 CFR, 46.406). Research conducted with children must, however, always be aimed at benefiting children rather than adults.

Ensuring that studies with children are scientifically valid

To be ethical, a research project involving children has to be well designed and well conducted and employ the minimum number of subjects (allowing for withdrawals) consistent with obtaining statistically valid results. The British Paediatric Association guidelines (BPA 1992, p.11) emphasise that: 'since the assessment of potential benefits and harm is so complex, children are best protected if projects are reviewed at many levels by researchers, funding and scientific bodies, local medical research ethics committees, the research assistants and nurses working with subjects, the children and their parents'.

But are all projects actually reviewed at several levels? For example in the UK, when a project is funded by an organisation such as the Medical Research Council, its scientific validity will have been carefully scrutinised by expert referees before funding was granted, but when research is financed out of departmental funds, it cannot always be assumed that it will have undergone the same external scrutiny. As mechanisms of peer review are developed, as is currently happening within teaching hospital National Health Service Trusts in the UK, the situation is likely to improve. Regardless of the method of funding, all proposals for research with children must be reviewed and approved by an ethics committee before they can go ahead. If the committee does not include experts in the field capable of assessing the project's scientific validity, where adequate peer review has not taken place, they should seek external advise. In considering studies on children, ethics committees should also seek advice from people with a close, practical knowledge of babies and children (e.g., a children's ward nurse or a paediatrician) to assess any potential distress that might be caused by the research. These advisors can already be ethics committee members, persons co-opted, members of a sub-committee or external advisors.

Risks and benefits

In order to assess whether any potential physical or psychological harm could result from the research, committee members will need to ask: (a) how invasive or intrusive is it?; (b) if there is a slight risk of harm, how likely is it to occur and how severe will the harm be?; and (c) will any harm be brief or long lasting and will it be immediately obvious or not evident until years later?

Low risk procedures

Acceptable low risk procedures include non-invasive scanning (Chapter 6) and questioning and observing children, provided that they are carried out in a sensitive manner and that consent has been given.

It does not follow that procedures routinely carried out in adults will be regarded as acceptable in children. For example, the insertion of a needle into the arm for injection or obtaining blood samples would be unlikely to raise any objections from an ethics committee as part of a study in adults. Although it may be regarded as having minimal risk in children (RCP 1996 s.8.6), many children fear needles, and multiple additional needle pricks in younger children are not acceptable unless there is the prospect of direct benefit to the child. If blood is required, when feasible it should be arranged with colleagues to withdraw small extra amounts into a syringe when samples are already being taken for diagnostic or treatment purposes. While venepuncture can be regarded as carrying only minimal risk when sterile disposable equipment is always used, risks could be unacceptable in parts of the world where conditions are less than ideal.

Higher risk procedures

Higher risks associated with new treatments may be acceptable when children are suffering from a dangerous disease, so long as the risk is no greater than that of the treatment the child would normally receive or, if none were available, of the risk of no treatment (CIOMS/WHO 1993, g.5). In such cases the harm to the child needs to be carefully assessed, so that all avoidable distress resulting from their condition, medical treatment and taking part in the research, may be prevented.

High risk procedures such as lung or liver biopsy, arterial puncture and cardiac catheterisation are not justified for research purposes and should only be carried out when essential for the diagnosis or treatment of the child.

Psychological damage

In research with children concern must not only be for the possibility of physical harm but also for the risk of any social and psychological effects. Indeed, few researchers would contemplate carrying out research with children if there was a risk of physical harm unless their condition was so serious that it was a question of survival. More frequently we are talking about psychological and social damage – in particular, that which might arise from breaches of confidentiality.

Confidentiality

The BPA emphasises the duty of the researcher to respect confidentiality, and to keep up to date with data protection and legislation on access to health records. Maintaining confidentiality is often considered of less importance where children are concerned than for adults, but in my view it is often more important. The slightest hint of being different in any way can result in a child being shunned, poked fun at or bullied at school. Take as an example, a study to assess the effects of very low birth weight on learning ability by the time the child reaches primary school. The researchers may find it convenient to conduct the assessments in the school, but how can this possibly be done without informing the teachers of the background of the study, and hence changing their perception of the child? What impression will the child's classmates get when the child is singled out for testing by a doctor who comes into the school?

Children are also entitled to have their confidence respected in regard to their parents (DoH 1996a). They may not, for instance, wish their parents to know that they are receiving counselling and would not want their parents to be approached for consent to participate in a research project where this was involved.

Issues relating to confidentiality are discussed more fully in Chapter 7.

Diagnosis of late onset diseases

Particularly difficult issues are raised by the early diagnosis in children of genetic predisposition to diseases that may not manifest themselves until later in life. Diagnosis of such conditions in children before the disease becomes apparent, might in a few cases enable treatment to be started early, but it may also adversely affect the child's self-perception, job prospects and freedom of choice. See Chapter 16 for a fuller discussion of the ethical issues associated with genetic testing in children.

Children should not be imposed upon

It is undesirable for children to be asked to participate in project after project simply because they happen to be available, or are much sought after because they have a rare illness, or one that is currently popular with researchers. It is hardly fair to impose on children who already have many problems. Older children who are capable of informed consent should normally be chosen in preference to younger, unless there are important scientific reasons for involving younger children (CIOMS/WHO 1993, g.5). Investigators are recommended to obtain the advice of the child's family physician on matters concerning their involvement in the research (BPA 1992, p.5; CIOMS/WHO 1993, g.5). When it is intended to contact the parents of young children for their participation in a study, particularly when this concerns the physical and intellectual development of children who suffered problems in the neonatal period or early infancy, care should be taken to establish from the family doctors that all of the children are still alive before contacting their parents.

In hospital-based research, care should be taken to ensure that the extra demands of the research do not filter staff away from the care of other children, or significantly delay access to diagnostic or other equipment for patients not in the study.

Assessment of potential benefits

To assess how great the benefits are likely to be, both the severity of the disease and how common the problem is, have to be taken into account. Questions to be addressed include: how likely is the research to achieve its aims; is it intended to benefit the subjects and/or other children; will potential benefits be limited because they are very expensive, or require specially trained professionals or a high input of time and effort? This last consideration should not of course stop work from being carried out.

Research with children should not simply duplicate earlier work. To avoid any unnecessary duplication, the development of databases not only of published but also of unpublished research should be encouraged to help researchers keep up-to-date with what is going on in other centres.

Acknowledging the time and effort put in by the children and their parents

Families should never be offered any financial inducement for their child's participation (CPMP 1997, s.1.1; 45 CFR). Participation in a study can, however, involve considerable time and effort on the part of children and their parents. Does it mean that time will have to be taken off school and work, or will very early morning visits to a clinic have to be made to avoid this? Will expenses be paid? As part of the informed consent procedure, investigators must explain clearly, both verbally and in the participant information sheet, prior to enrolment, exactly what will be involved.

Travelling expenses should always be paid if, for example, extra visits to clinics have to be made for the purposes of the research, although not if the research takes place in the course of a routine clinic visit which would have been made anyway. Patients should always be encouraged to accept travelling expenses as a routine and not be put in the embarrassing situation of having to ask for them. The provision of refreshments is especially important where children are concerned, not only for the participants themselves, but for any other children the parents may have had to bring along. Although payment is not appropriate, for young children balloons, badges and stickers and for older children vouchers to exchange at a bookshop or record store, may be given as a token of appreciation.

Are pure cost effectiveness studies in children unethical?

The BPA takes the view that research with children is not justifiable if undertaken primarily for financial advantage (BPA 1992, p.4). If this statement were to be taken as referring to the financial advantage of institutions as well as that of individual researchers it would appear to rule out cost effectiveness studies involving children, except perhaps where the cost element is only a minor part of the project. While such studies may be permissible in adults who freely give informed consent, it seems over optimistic to assume that many children would be so concerned with the financial management of the health service as to be willing to submit to discomfort in order to help their local hospital save some money.

Establish whether the child will be able to continue receiving the treatment at the end of the study

What will happen at the end of the study must be established at the outset. When it concerns a drug that has already been licensed for use in adults, if the child participants found it to be beneficial and still needed it at the end of the trial, would they be offered it? Is it possible that the health authority or hospital might decide it was too expensive for them to purchase? If they did, would the sponsor then be prepared to supply it free of charge? In the case of a drug for which the granting of a product licence is imminent, will it be possible to continue giving it on a 'named patient basis'?

In some types of research, continuing to provide the treatment at the end of the trial may pose a considerable financial burden not only to a pharmaceutical company but also to a hospital, independent researchers or parents. Computer technology, for instance, has led to the development of a variety of learning aids for children with learning difficulties, which involve the use of expensive computers in school and the loan of equipment for use at home. But what will happen at the end of the study? Will the child's 'toy' suddenly be taken away? Of particular concern is the situation where the equipment turns out to be more than just a toy and is found to be making a positive contribution to the child's development and well-being. Will the parents be able to purchase the equipment at an affordable price or will it be made available in the long-term from research funds?

Researchers should adequately address this aspect before embarking on the study and make the situation clear to prospective participants and their parents both verbally and in the information sheets.

Obtaining informed consent from children and their parents

The principles of informed consent discussed at length in Chapter 4 apply as much to studies with children as to those with adults, the difference being that some children will be too young to consent on their own behalf. The child's written consent should be obtained where feasible, but their willing co-operation (*assent*) should *always* be obtained (DoH 1991, s.4.4; BPA 1992, p.13; CIOMS/WHO 1993, g.5; RCP 1996, s.8.4). One possible exception to this is identified in the US regulations (45 CFR, 46.408) where the intervention holds out a prospect of direct benefit to the health of the children that is available only in the context of the research. In such cases full approval of the ethics committee must first be obtained. Apart from this rare exception, if a child objects to the research he or she should not be forced to participate.

In obtaining consent from children, the stage of development and degree of understanding of the child rather than their chronological age should be taken into account. Thus a child as young as seven may be able to understand the nature of some kinds of research if carefully explained. A child's ability to understand the nature of the research, like an adult's, as well as depending on its complexity will also depend on whether or not the child is already familiar, as a result of their illness, with the proposed methods. A young child with diabetes or haemophilia is likely to understand more about their illness and its treatment than the average non-affected adult. Children should be fully informed about the study in language and terms that they are able to understand. A simplified patient information sheet comprehensible to children of the age being recruited should be provided in addition to that for parents and older children.

If the children are insufficiently mature to consent on their own behalf, the consent of the parents must be obtained. It is advisable to obtain the consent of both parents when practicable, both for ethical reasons and to avoid the danger of the researcher later being confronted by an irate second parent raising objections to research being carried out on their child about which they were not consulted. The American regulations state that when more than minimal risk is involved unless the research is expected to be of direct benefit to the child both parents must give their consent. Exceptions to this rule are where one parent is unknown, not reasonably available or where only one parent has legal responsibility for the child (45 CFR, 46.408b).

There are rare circumstances in which the institutional review board may deem that parental consent is not appropriate, for example when an older child wishes to keep the nature of the treatment, such as counselling or treatment for a sexually transmitted disease, from their parents, or in cases of neglected or abused children (45 CFR, 46.408c).

The legal age of consent

This differs between countries. The Scottish Office guidance to ethics committees states: 'The Age of Legal Capacity (Scotland) Act 1991 provides that young people aged 16 and over in Scotland have full capacity to consent to examination or treatment on their own behalf. A child under the age of 16 is also capable of giving valid legal consent to a medical procedure or treatment (including research) provided he or she is, in the opinion of the qualified medical practitioner attending him/her, capable of understanding the nature and possible consequences of the procedure or treatment' (Scottish Office 1992). In practice, except in the rarest of circumstances, consent given by a child under 16 should, with the child's permission, be confirmed by the parent or guardian. Their consent, however, should not override the child's refusal to co-operate.

In England and Wales, children of 16 years and over can consent on their own behalf without parental approval to medical treat-ment (Family Law Reform Act 1969). In relation to research, the sit-uation is less clear cut, as the 1969 Act applies only to medical treatment (which some authorities believe may be taken to include therapeutic research) but not to non-therapeutic research. There is thus no precise age below 18 at which a child acquires legal capac-ity to consent to research. The validity of consent will therefore again depend on the child's understanding and intelligence (Medical Research Council 1991a; Grubb, 1997).

Despite the ethical requirement to obtain consent from parents or guardians, it should be emphasised that consent given by parents or guardians for their children to take part in research does not necessarily have any legal standing. If a child patient were later to bring an action against a researcher for injury suffered in the course of a research project, it would be a poor defence to say that informed consent had been obtained from the next of kin.

Parents must not give consent if they feel that it is against the child's interests

Parents have a responsibility not to give consent to research if they consider it to be against their child's interests, no matter how much obligation they feel under to agree. They can consent to research on a child if the research is designed to be of direct benefit to the child, but if that is not the case, they must only consent if the risks are so small that the research cannot be said to go against the child's interests (BPA 1992, p.12).

Also pressure should not be exerted on families by allowing them to feel guilty or ungrateful if they do not participate. They should be given sufficient time – several days if possible – to decide whether to participate and to discuss the project with their family doctor if they wish. It should not follow that because an ethics committee raises no ethical objections to a study, the parent or child should feel obliged to take part in it. If they consider that the project will cause too much disruption, discomfort or distress for *them*, they must say so. They are the ones involved and the final decision must be theirs.

The right to withdraw

In seeking informed consent, the researcher must make it clear to the child and to the parents that participation is entirely voluntary and that they may refuse to participate or can withdraw from the study at any stage, even after they have signed a consent form and taken part in the first phase. They must be assured that they do not have to give a reason for withdrawing and that the child's continued treatment will not be affected as a result (45 CFR 46).

Parents should be encouraged to stay with their child during the research so that they can withdraw the child if they consider it in their child's best interest (CIOMS/WHO 1993, g.5). Researchers must be available to respond to the family's questions and concerns throughout the study. Children should also be constantly monitored for signs of anxiety or distress, which may necessitate their withdrawal from the study by the researchers themselves (BPA 1992, p.11).

All studies involving children should be subject to regular monitoring by the ethics committee. See under 'Further reading' for other publications relating to research with children.

Seriously ill patients

It may not always be possible to obtain the consent of seriously ill patients, such as those who have suffered a heart attack, stroke or serious injury, for their entry into a research project aimed at determining the best treatment and, if consent is to be obtained, the only option may be to seek it from relatives. As the law stands in the UK, no one is empowered to give consent on behalf of another adult (DoH 1996a), in the sense that if the patient was injured by the research and sued the hospital, a relative's consent would not carry the same weight as would that of the patient's consent. Despite the legal uncertainties, the researcher would be expected from an ethical viewpoint to seek, whenever possible, the consent of a patient's next of kin.

Is it fair to ask relatives to consent?

It has to be acknowledged, however, that successfully obtaining consent from relatives in itself raises important ethical issues. Is it really fair to impose such a heavy burden on the relatives of seriously ill patients by asking them to consent to research on their behalf? Even if they are available, their distressed condition and the need for an instant decision goes against the likelihood of their consent being informed. What if the patient should die or suffer permanent injury during the study. Even though the injury may be totally unrelated to the study, a relative may be left with a feeling of guilt, wondering whether, if they had refused, their relative might still be alive.

If treatment has to be initiated immediately, it will often be the case that no relative is available to give consent. Must such patients be excluded from the trial?

Can research be done on seriously ill patients without consent from anyone?

Most official guidelines are vague and noncommittal on this issue. The US report (Office for Protection from Research Risks 1996) which lays down the conditions which must be met before research can go ahead on this basis is therefore welcome. These conditions are summarised below.

- The patients are in a life-threatening situation, available treatments are unproven or unsatisfactory, and the collection of valid scientific evidence is necessary to determine the effectiveness and safety of particular interventions.
- Obtaining informed consent is not feasible because:
  - (a) the patients will not be able to give informed consent as a result of their condition;
  - (b) the intervention involved in the research must be administered before consent from the patient's next of kin is feasible;
  - (c) there is no reasonable way to identify prospectively the individuals likely to become eligible for participation in the research.
- Participation in the research holds out the prospect of direct benefit to the patients because:
  - (a) patients are facing a life-threatening situation that necessitates intervention;
  - (b) appropriate animal and/or pre-clinical studies have been conducted, and the information supports the potential for the intervention to provide direct benefit;
  - (c) risks associated with the research are reasonable in relation to what is known about the medical condition and the risks of standard therapy.
- The research protocol defines the period in which treatment must be initiated and that every effort is made to obtain consent from relatives within this period.
- The institutional review board, (or in the UK, the local medical research ethics committee) must have given its approval to the project
- An independent data monitoring committee should be set up to exercise oversight of the research.

The above conditions do not appear particularly controversial and may form the basis of an international standard.

The report goes on to require that, in order to achieve further protection of the rights and welfare of the subjects, the intention to carry out the study should be publicly disclosed to the communities in which it will be conducted and from which the patients will be drawn. The researchers should also consult with representatives of those communities, and at the end of the study the results of the research should be made freely available. This is an extremely interesting idea and worthy of careful consideration, although it is not an approach that is often taken with such studies in the UK.

Legal constraints must not be allowed to prevent research into serious conditions from taking place

Refusal by the legal profession to allow the enrolment of seriously ill patients in research without consent would mean that certain categories of potentially life-saving research could never be carried out. It would make it impossible to establish which are the most effective methods of resuscitation, to develop new drugs for dissolving blood clots or to limit the area of damage in the brain immediately following a stroke.

To subject patients to research without their consent or that of a relative is clearly a very serious matter and can only be allowed if the design of the study is of proven scientific validity, and if there is a likelihood of direct benefit to the patient group concerned. The strictest scientific review by expert referees and careful scrutiny by a properly constituted ethics committee is required before such research can be allowed to proceed.

Patients with learning disability, serious psychiatric problems and all forms of dementia

Learning disability

In the past, persons with learning disability were sometimes chosen as research subjects perhaps because they were less capable of understanding what was to be done to them and less likely to object. This cannot be allowed to happen today.

In the case of children with learning disability the principles which apply to all children should be followed (RCP 1990b, s.7.35). People with learning disability should never be invited to participate in research that can be done equally well with volunteers or patients able to give informed consent (RCP 1990b, s.7.36; CIOMS/WHO 1993, g.6). This excludes knowingly recruiting persons with learning disability into a study, for example, of diabetes just because they happen to turn up at a clinic during the recruitment phase. People with learning disability may, however, be given the opportunity to participate in certain kinds of research if its purpose is to obtain knowledge relevant to their particular health needs (RCP 1990b, s.7.36; CIOMS/WHO 1993, g.6).

There are certain conditions which affect only persons with learning disability. For example, in Rett's syndrome (a condition that affects about one in 10,000 females) air swallowing occurs in about half of patients with the illness. It is distressing both for patients and their carers, and can be dangerous because of the possibility of the high pressures generated damaging the gastrointestinal tract. Because of the dangers associated with air swallowing, it would not be ethically acceptable to encourage volunteers to do it deliberately and the research can, therefore, only be done with patients who swallow air as part of their condition.

There are also medical conditions that can affect anyone but where persons with learning disability may benefit most from improvements in treatment. A familiar example is tooth decay. Consider a trial to compare the acceptability of the conventional method of removing decay from a tooth using a drill and the recently introduced method using a laser. Dental drills tend to be noisy and as there has to be contact between the rotating bur and the tooth, vibration is unavoidable. As people with learning disability are amongst those most likely to be to put off seeking regular dental treatment because of this, it would make sense to include them in a trial to see if they find the new laser method more acceptable.

Although the official guidelines appear not to offer any advice on this, where persons with learning disability stand to benefit more than the general population, it may be considered acceptable to offer them the chance of participating. This can only be done so long as the procedure or new drug being tested has previously been shown to carry no more than minimal risk in healthy volunteers and normal patients, and with the prior approval of the ethics committee. It has to be recognised, however, that some studies, such as those using intrusive questionnaires or high-tech training methods involving immersion in a virtual environment (e.g. for road traffic training), while not raising any ethical issues when conducted in healthy volunteers, may do so if conducted with persons with learning disability, in whom extra care must be taken to avoid causing confusion or alarm, or raising uncertainties.

Many proposals for research with persons with learning disability are of a psychological or social nature, designed to benefit them as a group. These may include studies such as comparing methods of training to cross the road safely, which require ethical approval only because participants are selected as persons with a particular medical condition.

Avoiding exploitation of persons with learning disability

One group of patients currently in considerable demand as research subjects are those with Down's Syndrome. The association of Down's Syndrome with a number of other medical conditions makes them potential subjects for researchers in several different specialities. While this typically means no more than the donation of small blood samples, care should be taken to ensure that they are not subjected to too much unwelcome attention.

Obtaining consent from persons with learning disability

There are many different kinds and degrees of learning disability and many patients, depending on the extent of the disability, will be able to give consent on their own behalf. Ensuring that the consent is informed may be more difficult and require special skills and patience in putting over the information, but it should be attempted whenever possible. If patients cannot give consent on their own behalf, a relative should be consulted and their consent given, even if this does not have any standing in the law of the country concerned (RCP 1990b, s.7.40). Even if patients can give consent, it is advisable for it to be witnessed by a relative. Although they may not be able to give informed consent, the willing co-operation of people with learning disability to take part in the research should always be sought, and any objections on their part respected. (CIOMS/WHO 1993, g.6).

Serious psychiatric problems

Research with psychiatric patients is as essential as with any other kind of patient if new validated methods of treatment are to be established. Not to allow psychiatric patients to become involved in research would be unethical, as this is the only way they are going to obtain improved treatments for, and insight into, their condition. As with other vulnerable groups, research should only be done with patients known to have serious psychiatric problems if it cannot be done with otherwise healthy adults, and it must be specifically aimed at benefiting patients with such problems. Apart from this, most of the ethical issues raised by research with psychiatric patients are those raised by medical research in general. Most patients, despite their illness, will be capable of discussing the proposal with the researcher and deciding whether or not to give informed consent and participate.

Confidentiality

Owing to the stigma that unfortunately still tends to be attached to psychiatric illness, the preservation of strict confidentiality is as important as with research into most medical problems. The strict rules of confidentiality discussed in Chapter 7 must therefore always be adhered to. Difficulties may arise if, in the course of a study, information is unexpectedly obtained which should be passed on, such as if patients reveal that they are suicidal or intend to harm someone. In studies where such revelations are remotely possible, the researcher should normally make it clear to the patients at the outset that any information considered important for their medical care will be passed on to their family doctor or consultant. This should be repeated both verbally and in the information sheet, and consent to do so obtained.

Many studies do not start out with psychiatric patients, but are designed to identify those with psychiatric illness within certain groups, such as depression amongst people suffering from an incurable illness like motor neurone disease or caring for relatives with serious brain injuries, or amongst overworked medical staff. This often involves the completion of standard diagnostic questionnaires. Participants must always be told at the outset, as part of the informed consent procedure, if it is the intention to inform their family doctor or a psychiatrist if they register a certain critical score, or indeed if it is the intention to inform the participants.

Studies to identify members of certain groups suffering psychiatric problems should not be conducted in a vacuum as an academic exercise simply to estimate incidence. Arrangements should always be made to offer medical help or counselling for those found to be affected, if they want it.

Special problems with obtaining freely informed consent in psychiatric studies

A special problem with some kinds of psychiatric research is that by making the patient fully aware of the design of the study it may influence the behaviour or attitudes which it is aimed to measure. For example, a typical study aimed at assessing the patients' reactions to different forms of therapy – group therapy, regular one-to-one therapy with a counsellor, or less frequent sessions with a trained psychiatrist – where knowledge that another group of patients was receiving a different level of help from themselves might well influence a patient's response. In studies of this type, where patients need to be allocated to a group without being told of the existence of others, they should be informed that there are certain facts which cannot be revealed now as this might influence the results, but which will be revealed at the end of the study.

The key question to be addressed by an ethics committee is whether knowledge of the information that is not revealed would have prevented the patient from taking part in the study. If it would have done so, the study should not be allowed to go ahead (Royal College of Psychiatrists 1990).

Some psychiatric patients, as a result, for example, of anxiety or depression, may find it difficult to concentrate sufficiently on the information being provided in order to understand it fully enough to be able to give informed consent. Great care must be taken by researchers in such circumstances to ensure that the consent they obtain is valid.

Psychiatric patients may be even more prone than most other groups of patient to perceive a need to please the doctor who has already helped or might help them in the future. While medical outpatients may see a different member of the medical team almost every time they attend the clinic, in psychiatric care the building up of a trusting doctor–patient relationship is often seen as an essential part of the treatment. It is important therefore, for the researcher, especially if the researcher is also the patients' doctor, to emphasise that participation is entirely voluntary and that they may refuse to participate or withdraw from the study later without giving a reason and without it affecting their future medical care or relationship with the staff.

The prospect of extra attention may also be a powerful inducement to participate.

Psychiatric researchers, therefore, have a special responsibility to ensure that patients do not feel under any sort of pressure to take part.

Detained patients

Where a patient is detained in hospital for treatment without consent under the appropriate mental health legislation of the country concerned (e.g., in the UK, the Mental Health Act 1983), the question arises as to the situation regarding consent to research. There is a fundamental difference between the position of the detained patient and that of other members of the community in that patients who are not detained have the right *not* to receive treatment, whereas the detained patient on admission to hospital losses the right not to receive treatment. A position paper produced by the Mental Health Act Commission (1997) takes the view that detained patients may, in the case of therapeutic research forming an essential part of their treatment, be given an experimental drug which it is believed will be of benefit to them without their consent. No such study is allowed to go ahead, however, without the approval of an independent research ethics committee. The initial phase I testing of a new drug should already have been conducted in healthy volunteers. An important point here is that the use of placebo in a clinical trial would undermine the reason for the patient's detention, which was to provide compulsory treatment, and would not be acceptable. This limits the kind of clinical trial that can be carried out with detained patients. In regard to non-therapeutic research, there is clearly no justification for not obtaining informed consent from detained patients, and the requirements for obtaining their fully informed consent, without coercion, prior to participation will be essentially the same as for other patients (Anon 1997a; Mental Health Act Commission 1997).

Dementia

In common with other vulnerable groups, patients with dementia must only be recruited into studies directly related to their condition. This raises the question of how, when someone turns up at say a diabetic clinic, does the researcher know whether the patient has mild learning disability or is in the early stages of dementia? The administration of tests to assess cognitive functioning (which include simple questions such as: 'what day is it?'; 'spell *world* backwards') might cause offence if done routinely. It may, however, be acceptable to administer them in a situation where a significant proportion of patients will need to be excluded, as in research conducted with elderly patients in a long-stay ward.

As emphasised by the Alzheimer's Disease Society (1993), Alzheimer's disease is a condition for which advances in knowledge and treatment are desperately needed. Progress towards finding the causes and developing new approaches to treatment will only be possible so long as people with the condition and their relatives and carers are willing to participate in research.

Taking care to avoid raising false hopes

When a project is basic research with no possibility of immediate therapeutic benefit, investigators must ensure that relatives and, as far as their condition allows, patients with dementia are fully aware that they themselves are unlikely to benefit directly from participation. They must be aware that it is being carried out in order to develop methods of prevention and treatment so that people may benefit in the future. Many patients with dementia and their relatives, on realising this, are pleased to volunteer out of the feeling that, through their own misfortune, they may be able to help others.

There is a danger that relatives of patients with dementia may come forward for drug trials in the belief that they may be the first in line for a wonder drug. They are almost certain to be disappointed. There have been drugs developed, notably antibiotics, that have provided a complete cure for specific diseases. The changes in the brain of a dementia sufferer, however, are very complex and few researchers believe that there can be such a straightforward cure, particularly as, by the time it is diagnosed, much damage has probably already been done. Great care must therefore be taken to avoid raising false hopes. There is real hope, nevertheless, that drugs may be developed that will alleviate symptoms or slow down the progression of the disease, particularly if detected early, and research is currently in progress with these aims.

Obtaining consent from patients with Alzheimer's disease and their relatives

It does not follow that someone with Alzheimer's disease or other form of dementia is incapable of deciding whether or not they wish to participate in a research project. The severity of the condition typically varies from day-to-day, and most patients will still be capable of expressing a view on whether or not they wish to participate. Indeed much of the current research on Alzheimer's disease focuses on the early phase of the condition when the patient may still be capable of giving consent to participation.

As there will, nevertheless, always be some doubt as to whether the consent of a patient with dementia is truly informed, the consent of a relative should also be obtained. As discussed in regard to research with children and persons with learning disability, consent by a third party does not necessarily have any standing in law. In the unlikely event of the researcher being sued by the patient, the fact that consent had been obtained from a relative may well be considered irrelevant. Despite this, it is essential from an ethical viewpoint, and whenever possible, consent must be sought from a close relative. Whatever the degree of dementia, patients should, as far as possible, be made aware of what will be involved. If not willing to participate in the research, then they should not be recruited, even if it is the relatives' wish that they should participate.

Maintaining confidentiality

Researchers should, however, take great care when approaching relatives of patients with dementia for consent, not to reveal confidential information. Whenever possible, non-visiting relatives should only be approached with the agreement of the patient. This is especially important if there is any possibility that the relative, who may be living elsewhere, is not aware of the patient's illness and the patient may not wish them to be presented with the diagnosis.

If the patient has no relatives

In basic research that is unlikely to be of any direct benefit, it might seem prudent to exclude the patient from the study when there is no relative available to give consent. In a trial of a new, potentially beneficial drug, however, it would be unfair to exclude patients from receiving a treatment which might be of benefit to them simply because they did not have a relative to support their wish to be included. When there is no relative available, a carer may be appointed instead. The type of carer who can be asked to consent on behalf of a person with Alzheimer's disease needs to be clarified. While a long-standing friend might qualify, it is doubtful whether a member of staff of a nursing home which the patient has only just entered should be expected to shoulder this responsibility.

13

Research on surplus blood and other tissue

So far, the main government regulations and professional guidelines fail to deal adequately with the ethical issues involved in the use of spare tissue. Research that involves absolutely no physical risk or discomfort to patients but simply takes advantage of 'left over' blood or other tissue appears uncontroversial and is an obvious candidate for expedited review/chairperson's action. Are there, therefore, any ethical pitfalls?

When taking blood samples, it is common practice to draw slightly more than is strictly required for the diagnostic tests to be performed. This saves having to return to the patient to insert another needle should the test have to be repeated. Similarly when removing cancerous or other diseased tissue, it is usual also to take some surrounding tissue, as a precaution. The surplus may be deep frozen and stored for future reference. Other potential sources of human tissue include that removed at hysterectomy, or in reducing the obstruction caused by an enlarged prostate gland and, of course, the placenta.

Must patients' permission be obtained?

Most people (so long as their religion does not forbid it) are only too willing to allow their own body fluids to be used to help others. Millions donate blood to replace that which others have lost following injury or surgery, or for the extraction of proteins for treating patients with conditions such as haemophilia. Why then should anyone object if spare blood is used for research that is aimed at obtaining information of benefit to future generations of patients?

If extra blood or tissue is to be removed specifically for research, the patient will clearly need to give consent. When, however, patients are not being subjected to any extra risks, discomfort or inconvenience and when the tissue would normally be discarded, does the researcher even need to ask their permission before using it? If the patient hates reading and filling in forms, he or she may prefer that the doctor did not bother to ask.

Despite first impressions, a more detailed examination of the potential uses of spare tissue reveals that the situation is more complex than might appear.

Is the intended use of the tissue ethical?

Risks and discomforts to participants are not the only ethical issues that have to be considered. There is also the question of whether the uses to which it is intended to put the tissue might be considered unethical by some potential donors.

An anonymous study that employed cells scraped from the surface of the roots of teeth obtained by routine extraction, might not at first sight appear to pose any ethical problems or need to be referred to an ethics committee. This situation, however, would change if the cells were to be used for producing cell lines.

Cell and tissue culture

Most people would probably not object to their spare tissue being chopped up and enzymes or other components extracted from it, but the creation of cell lines is a potentially controversial issue. Cells from patients with a particularly interesting condition may be grown in culture so that they can be studied at will and passed to specialist researchers in other laboratories. The cell lines may be 'immortalised' giving them the potential for life decades after the patient who donated them is dead. Does it matter? The researcher and ethics committee may give an opinion, but only the individuals concerned can say whether this would be acceptable to them personally. When cell or tissue culture is involved, informed consent for the use of spare tissue is essential.

The question of the ownership of the cells, should it be wished to exploit the cell line commercially, also has to be addressed, although this is more of a financial than an ethical issue (Nuffield Council on Bioethics 1995, p.83–99).

Prenatal diagnosis and abortion

It may be reasonably assumed that a woman strongly opposed to abortion would not wish her placenta to be used to develop new agents of abortion. A researcher wishing to obtain a placenta for research must, therefore, explain to the patient exactly what it is to be used for so that, if she considers the use unethical, she can refuse consent. Blood and other tissues are often employed in research aimed at identifying the genes responsible for certain genetic disorders. When this information could lead to the prenatal diagnosis of genetic defects, and hence to parents of the future being given the option of aborting affected fetuses, patients opposed to abortion might well object to their spare tissue being used in this way. They must be made aware of the possibility of this outcome and be given the opportunity to say no. It must be made easy for them, for example by being able to tick a 'No' box on a form rather than having to inform an enthusiastic researcher of their unwillingness, face-to-face.

Transgenic animals

The creation of transgenic animals is another controversial use of spare human tissue. A human gene carrying the information for producing a hormone or other valuable protein, may be introduced into the cells of, for example, a living cow, so that the cow produces abundant amounts of the protein in its milk, from which it is then extracted. Some patients will object to their genes being used in this way on ethical grounds. There is again the question of ownership of body parts in the event of commercial exploitation of interesting pieces of DNA. Going one step further, the transplantation, not just of sections of DNA, but of pieces of spare tissue into animals, increases the likelihood of objections.

Patients and healthy volunteers must be told exactly what their spare blood or other tissue is to be used for, so that they have the opportunity to refuse to allow it to be used if they consider the researcher's aim to be unethical.

The detection of unexpected illness

Of major concern is how the results of research on spare tissue, particularly unexpected ones, may affect the patient. Imagine that spare blood from a patient was being used as a normal control in an experiment and, for the sake of the safety of the staff, underwent a routine test for HIV antibodies and was unexpectedly found to be HIV positive. This would create a serious dilemma for the doctor if the patient had not given permission for the blood to be used in this way. To avoid such situations arising in the first place, participants must be told exactly what new tests will be performed on their blood, whether the results could be traced back to them and, if so, what the procedure would be if an abnormality were detected. If it is intended to inform their family doctor of any unsuspected findings, participants must be prewarned of this intention and give their prior consent.

Genetic studies on archived tissues

Excess blood and biopsy material that have been deep frozen and stored for future reference provide a convenient source of tissue for researchers wanting to conduct basic biochemical or genetic studies thus avoiding the necessity of taking new biopsies. In the rare situation where the work is being done anonymously with no possibility of the results being traced back to the patients concerned and where there are no ethical issues involved, an ethics committee may consider it acceptable to use such tissue without patients' permission. If, however, there is a possibility of obtaining results of which patients or their family doctor should be informed, or if tissue culture, prenatal diagnosis or other ethical issues are involved, the permission of patients must be obtained before the stored blood or tissue is used.

As the list of known genetic mutations and gene variants associated with particular conditions increases, researchers are increasingly presented with the opportunity of testing samples of blood to determine whether there is a genetic element to the patient's illness.

Blood may have been taken during a previous non-genetic study for which consent and ethical approval was duly obtained, and stored in the deep freeze. Once a genetic test becomes available, it is tempting just to take these samples and test them. In Chapter 16 there is a fuller discussion of the ethics of this and other aspects of genetic screening.

Uses less likely to raise serious ethical issues

Improving existing diagnostic tests

Tissue taken for diagnostic tests is sometimes used in efforts to improve the reliability of those tests. Smears taken during routine screening for cervical cancer, for example, may also be used to devise improved methods of detecting pre-cancerous cells. If the smear used for the research is the same one as used for the standard test, the patient is not involved in any extra discomfort and no new knowledge of relevance to her is likely to arise, there are unlikely to be any ethical implications. Similarly, if blood is sent to a laboratory for measuring, for example the level of a hormone, there is no objection to the laboratory using what is left over to devise an improved method of measuring the same hormone. As the patient will already know from the standard test what their hormone level is, the possibility of abnormal findings of which the patient or the family doctor would need to be made aware does not exist.

These are rare exceptions to the rule that informed consent and ethical approval must be obtained before spare blood and other tissue can be used in research. Even in this type of activity, however, ethical implications could still arise if performing the new test were to result in a delay in providing the results of the standard test. If this possibility existed, the patient's informed consent would first have to be obtained.

Calibration of equipment for standard tests

Extra or unused blood, saliva or other materials are needed to calibrate laboratory tests and equipment. If the doctor wishes to take a few extra millilitres of blood for calibration purposes into a syringe already inserted to withdraw blood for clinical reasons it is sufficient to tell the patient and obtain verbal consent. Verbal agreement will also be sufficient if blood is taken from healthy volunteers for calibration of laboratory equipment, so long as there is no possibility of serious abnormal findings.

Tissue samples may also be stored for quality control purposes, as in the storage of cervical smears, to enable periodic checks to be made on the accuracy of the original examinations, but this is medical audit rather than research and is unlikely to raise ethical issues.

Is the tissue really spare?

When it is stated that only spare tissue is to be used for research, it really must be spare. The ethics committee scrutinising a proposal to use spare tissue will need assurance that in, for example, a study using spare skin obtained at routine surgery, no additional skin will be taken for the purpose of the study. To reduce the risk of this happening, ideally the surgeon removing the tissue should not be directly involved in the research project.

It is also essential that apparently spare tissue is only used for research after it has been established that it will not be needed for histological or other clinical examination.

Summary

In view of the many ethical issues raised by research on spare blood and other tissue, the rule is, with very few exceptions, that the donor's informed consent should be obtained before such material is used for research purposes. There are a number of questions to which donors will require answers: (a) what is the blood/tissue being used for; (b) could the results be traced back to the donor; (c) would the results be reported to the donor's family doctor; (d) if so, could the results have any consequences for employment or insurance; (e) is the blood to be stored; and (f) if so, will the donor be consulted before it is used for any other purpose?

Proposed guidelines for consent for the use of spare blood and other tissues

In the absence of official guidelines on the subject, the following are proposed:

(1) Consent need not be obtained if spare blood/tissue is used to calibrate instruments, so long as there is no possibility of abnormal findings relevant to the donor.

(2) Consent need not be obtained if spare blood/tissue is used to evaluate a new test for a factor for which a standard test already exists, so long as:
    (a) the patient already knows the result of the standard test;
    (b) there is no possibility of new findings relevant to the patient.

(3) Verbal consent will be needed if *extra* blood, swabs, etc. have to be taken for (1) or (2) above.

(4) Informed written consent must be obtained for genetic or other testing of fresh or stored blood/tissue, which is not done anonymously, when the results may be relevant to the participants or their relatives (*even when this means contacting again participants for consent several years after the sample was taken*).

(5) Informed written consent will be required for the use of spare blood/tissue if there are ethical issues involved (regardless of whether or not the results are relevant to the participants). Ethical issues will arise if it is used for:

   (a) the development of agents of abortion;

   (b) the development of methods of pre-natal testing that might result in the decision to abort affected fetuses testing positive (*even if the research is at an early stage and involves only the use of samples of blood from a random population*);

   (c) cell or tissue culture;

   (d) the transfer of tissue or genetic material into other persons or animals.

(6) Verbal consent for the use of spare blood/tissue is acceptable so long as:

   (a) none of the ethical issues in (4) or (5), or other ethical issues, apply;

   (b) the samples are tested anonymously, with no possibility of them being linked to the donor.

(7) If it is intended to communicate abnormal findings to the patient's family doctor or other party, prior consent must be given for this.

(8) Consent for *unspecified* future use of stored blood/tissue is not acceptable.

In view of the potential ethical issues raised by proposals for research on spare blood and other tissue, approval by an ethics committee must be sought before the research can go ahead. An exception to this rule may be made in the case of the situations outlined in points (1) to (3) above.

14

Questionnaire and interview studies

Studies which involve no more than the administration of a questionnaire or a structured interview, might appear at first sight unlikely to raise any ethical concerns that would necessitate scrutiny by a full medical research ethics committee. Even if requiring to be submitted to an ethics committee at all, it would seem that most could be dealt with by chairperson's action. There is little official guidance on questionnaire studies. The Royal College of Physician's (1996, s.7.50–7.52) guidelines are exceptional in devoting as many as five sentences to their discussion.

Despite this lack of official interest, questionnaire studies have to be considered as seriously as other kinds of study, as many questionnaires have the potential for causing significant distress to those invited to complete them. The aim of this chapter is to highlight the ethical issues that may be raised by questionnaire studies, and to emphasise the care with which the questions posed need to be considered by the researcher and the ethics committee before being presented to participants.

Epidemiological questionnaires

Questionnaires are often used by epidemiologists to obtain the information required to initiate health education campaigns and to monitor whether the initiatives are working. They may be used to determine why people living in some areas are more prone to certain illnesses than those in others. 'What do you eat and how much exercise do you take?,' are typical of the questions asked. Participants are usually chosen at random. The questionnaires rarely cause offence or raise matters of confidentiality or any other ethical issues, although care has to be taken not to stigmatise people living in certain parts of town as, for example, being less healthy than those from other parts.

Quality of life questionnaires

There are other questionnaires, however, that ask more search-ing questions. Researchers often wish to compare how patients feel both physically and emotionally, before, during and after treat-ment. In order to collect this information, questionnaires are designed so that patients can complete them at various stages of their treatment. Such questionnaires typically refer to how well the patients have been feeling during the past week and are designed to monitor any side-effects they may be experiencing. Most of the questions will enquire about their physical condition: 'Have you felt nauseated?' or 'Have you had pain?', which most people would probably not regard as particularly confidential.

This changes when, as is often the case, a psychological ques-tionnaire is included asking questions of a more personal nature: 'Do you ever feel cheerful?'; 'Have you lost interest in your appear-ance?'; 'Do you get a sort of frightened feeling as if something awful is about to happen?', or even questions about sexual activity. Issues of confidentiality now begin to arise. If participants are to reply honestly to such questions, they must be confident that the infor-mation they give will be strictly confidential, and accessible only to the researchers and senior medical staff. Some patients may also feel intimidated by questions about their relationships and demand strict confidentiality before revealing, for example, who they are living with. In the interests of confidentiality, completed questionnaires should be identified by code number rather than using the participant's name.

Before   sending   questionnaires   to   named   participants, researchers must carefully consider whether they have a right to the participants' names and addresses. If the researcher has never been directly involved in their care, might the patient regard the arrival of a questionnaire as evidence of a breach of confidentiality? If there is a risk of this, when feasible the initial approach should be made by the patient's usual doctor.

Audit questionnaires

A familiar use of questionnaires in health services is as a tool to gain patients' views about the service they have received or are receiving, or even about the research in which they have been involved. These rarely have any ethical implications beyond, again, the requirement for strict confidentiality, with patients being reassured that the medical staff will not find out what they have been saying about them.

Audit questionnaires, however, are not always completely innocuous. A questionnaire issued as part of an audit to obtain pregnant women's views about maternity services, for instance, may include potentially distressing questions, such as if they have suffered a miscarriage in a previous pregnancy or had a termination following prenatal testing. Most importantly, in studies of this type, the greatest of care needs to be taken to ensure that questionnaires are not sent to women who have suffered a miscarriage or perinatal death in their current pregnancy.

Questionnaires that raise patients' expectations

Ethical implications also arise when there is a danger that by asking certain questions, patients' expectations may be increased. In a typical study of what elderly people think of the community services they receive, the researcher may ask questions such as:

► 'Do you ever see a district nurse?'
► 'If not, would you like to see one?'
► 'What other type of help would you like to see available?'

If this is purely a research project, the researcher has a responsibility to make it clear to participants at the outset that he or she is not in a position to directly influence the services the participants receive. The researcher can tell the patients that if it was felt that they would benefit from extra help the researcher could, with their permission, inform their family doctor, but that it would then be up to the doctor and the patient to take things further if it is appropriate.

Intrusive questions with significant ethical implications

Have you felt like attempting suicide?

As an example of a type of questionnaire that may have more serious ethical implications let us consider one administered to patients with a physical illness to identify those suffering from depression. Would it be acceptable to bombard patients with the following series of questions in rapid succession?

Have you recently:
- been thinking of yourself as a worthless person?;
- felt that life is entirely hopeless?;
- felt that life isn't worth living?;
- thought of the possibility that you might make away with yourself?;
- found at times you couldn't do anything because your nerves were too bad?;
- found yourself wishing you were dead and away from it all?;
- found that the idea of taking your own life kept coming into your mind?

If you were suffering from toothache you might laugh it off, but what about the patient with a serious progressive disease. It could be argued that the questions were suggestive and might result in someone doing serious harm to themselves. These questions do in fact appear in a well-known standard health questionnaire

(Goldberg 1981) and questions like them feature in several other standard questionnaires.

When the questions are intrusive and/or may cause distress, the participant's consent must be sought before sending the questionnaire to them (Royal College of Physicians 1996, s.7.51), and the fact that some of the questions may be distressing to some individuals should be explained in the preliminary letter.

That a questionnaire is said to be standard or established or validated for use in a clinical context must never be taken to imply that it is ethically acceptable for the all groups of patients to whom the questionnaire may be administered as part of a research project. It may have slipped in through the ethical net long ago, or have been intended for a restricted group of patients under certain defined conditions. Continued debate and monitoring is always necessary in such cases. Unfortunately it is not usually possible for an ethics committee to require individual questions to be omitted, as this is likely to invalidate the questionnaire, so it has to be an all or nothing decision.

It would seem prudent never to administer psychiatric questionnaires in a vacuum just to obtain figures of incidence, for example, as part of a student project. The person in charge of the research must always ensure that adequate psychiatric backup is available to offer help to patients found to be depressed or otherwise in need of help.

Questionnaires for the seriously ill

Many well-intentioned questionnaires are designed to determine the needs of patients with serious illnesses and their families. Although intended to elicit information on patients' ability to cope and on their feelings, questionnaires have the potential for causing distress to very vulnerable people.

In studies of this type, it is recommended that the following precautions be taken:

► In order to minimise any potential distress to patients and relatives, the researcher should obtain written agreement from the relevant doctor allowing the researcher to invite patients under their care to take part in the study.

► An introductory letter explaining the study, which points out, if applicable, the possibility that certain questions might be distressing, and a consent form should be given or sent out prior to the questionnaire.

► Patients who wish to participate should be asked to return the consent form within a certain period of time and to contact the researcher to discuss any concerns. Once consent is obtained the questionnaire may then be sent out.

► When a questionnaire is to be readministered at intervals it is important to check prior to each mailing with the patients' doctors that they are still living, to avoid causing distress to relatives by sending out questionnaires to deceased patients.

It is essential to ensure that the potential benefit of the knowledge derived from such studies justifies the disturbance they may cause to seriously ill patients.

Intrinsically distressing questionnaire studies

There is another type of questionnaire study that may, by its nature, cause distress, even when no individual question is particularly intrusive. An example of this would be a study to examine the possibility that work and other activities during pregnancy are related to premature birth and late miscarriages. Mothers who have suffered a miscarriage are sent a questionnaire asking how many hours a week they worked during each month of their pregnancy, the nature of their job, whether they drank alcohol or smoked, and so on.

While the aim of the project is laudable – to identify work practises associated with preterm labour, premature delivery and miscarriage and to produce recommendations aimed at reducing the incidence of these major health problems – it has to be appreciated that replying to such a questionnaire could cause some women considerable distress, awakening a sense of guilt that through their own behaviour they may somehow have been responsible for the miscarriage.

In this type of questionnaire study, independent scrutiny by an ethics committee is essential. The committee might in this case require that the questionnaire be completed in the presence of a qualified counsellor rather than being posted to women at home.

Questions suitable for some but not for others

In considering the acceptability of a questionnaire, the target audience must also be taken into account. Questions on sexual activity, for instance, may be acceptable for administering to normal adults but inappropriate for young children, or some persons with learning disability.

Is informed consent required for questionnaire studies?

Ethics committees will not always require written informed consent for questionnaire studies so long as the questions are non-intrusive and it is made clear that participation is entirely voluntary and that refusal to participate will not affect any future medical care or, if applicable, their relationship with the staff looking after the participants. Return of the questionnaire may be taken as implied consent in such cases.

The situation changes, however, when the questionnaire includes questions that may be intrusive or distressing, as in the earlier examples of studies aimed at identifying patients with depression, or at evaluating how those with serious illness are coping. In such studies a preliminary letter explaining the reason for the study and the possibility of finding some questions distressing should be sent to potential participants, and their written consent obtained, *before* issuing the questionnaire (Royal College of Physicians 1996, s.7.50–7.51).

The response to questions cannot always be predicted. Some questions may trigger distress in some patients but not in others. It is difficult for participants to know until they have seen the questionnaire whether it is acceptable to them or not. When it is intended to re-administer a potentially distressing questionnaire to the same patients at intervals during the course of their illness, they should be asked if they wish to continue, before giving them the questionnaire again.

Avoid exhausting the participant with too many questionnaires

Some researchers seem unable to resist the temptation to administer all of the questionnaires they have available. This raises the question of whether participants are going to be overburdened with the task of completing them all, possibly resulting in an inadequate response rate and of whether all of the data can be satisfactorily analysed. To assess the amount of time required to complete a set of questionnaires it is advisable to carry out a pilot study, or at least get friends who have not seen them to try them out first (if necessary, in private and destroying them afterwards to avoid revealing confidential information about themselves). If it is intended to administer several questionnaires to the same participants, the researcher should provide the ethics committee with the justification for this.

Arranging a home interview

If the questionnaire is to be administered as a structured interview conducted in the participant's own home, care must be taken to ensure that the interviewer is properly introduced first. This precaution applies to any interview study. Ideally the interviewer should be accompanied on the first visit by the participant's family doctor or someone else who is personally known to them. If this is not considered appropriate, a definite appointment should be made to avoid the possibility of elderly patients inadvertently letting an intruder into their home thinking it was the interviewer they had been told to expect at sometime during the week (or not letting the interviewer into their home because they thought he or she might be an intruder). The name of the interviewer should be conveyed to the participant in advance and identification should always be shown.

Questionnaire studies on the Internet

The distribution of questionnaires over the Internet may be extremely attractive in large scale studies, not least because of the substantial savings in stationery and postage, and the likelihood of a more rapid, if not higher, response rate. At present, for most studies the potential participants would represent too narrow a sector of the target population, but as access to the Internet increases, possibly in developed countries, to a level similar to that of telephone usage, there may be a proliferation of questionnaire studies conducted in this way.

Where a target population selected on the basis of computer literacy is not a huge problem, research on the Internet is already feasible. For example, take a study to compare the benefits of providing sufferers with two types of information about a particular illness. The comparison is between on screen standard text such as patients might normally receive on paper at a clinic visit and an interactive computer-based system providing customised (but not personalised) information. When patients log onto the website they are presented with an information sheet that tells them about the study, and that if they want to 'sign' the consent form and go further, they will be randomly allocated to receive one of two types of information, which they can access as and when they wish. They are told that at the end of six months they will be e-mailed a questionnaire about how their illness has been affecting them, to be completed on screen and returned electronically.

As Internet-based questionnaires are now upon us, some basic ground rules need to be established, taking regard of special issues raised by the use of the Internet rather than personal contact, or the postal service. As I am not aware of any official guidelines having yet been issued on this matter, a suggested code of conduct is presented below.

- ▶ On contacting the web page, potential participants should initially be provided with an on screen information sheet. This should give: details of the background to the study; what is involved for them personally; if applicable, that some of the questions may be intrusive; steps taken to ensure confidentiality; a contact number to obtain further information over the telephone; and any significant costs involved.
- ▶ Completion of a consent form must be a prerequisite to participating in the research, with access denied unless the consent form is correctly completed.
- ▶ The consent form must, as a minimum, record the participant's understanding that:
  - (a) any information provided is no substitute for consultation with their doctor who knows the history of their illness and personal circumstances;
  - (b) that it is essential to contact a qualified medical practitioner in the event of a worsening of their condition.
- ▶ Individual questions on the consent form must be responded to with a response such as 'Yes I understand this', typed character by character, rather than with just a click of the mouse.
- ▶ Confidentiality of participants must be strictly maintained. Respondents must not be asked to reveal their names. For anonymous studies the e-mail address will be sufficient, while if personal contact with respondents is required, codes must be used.
- ▶ To accommodate participants using a *shared* e-mail address in a library, school, shared flat, Internet Café, etc., they should be given the option of accessing the questionnaire themselves if they wish (e.g., in response to a reminder that appears when they access the website, such as 'please remember to request your questionnaire

on date') rather than having it posted automatically, with the risk of revealing to the other users that one of their number has the illness concerned.

► On completion of the research, a summary of the findings should be provided for participants as in the above point.

► Questionnaire studies conducted on the Internet must be approved by an ethics committee before commencement and before implementing changes, in the same way as other questionnaire studies.

(Note: While required ethically as evidence of consent, no pronouncement can be made about the legal validity of a consent form completed over the Internet until it is tested in the courts.)

If in doubt, seek the advice of the ethics committee

If in doubt about whether the approval of the local medical research ethics committee is required, the researcher should seek the advice of the committee before issuing the questionnaires. In most cases, apart from the most innocuous of audit studies, ethical approval, at least by chairperson's action, if not by the full committee, will be required.

Before approving a proposal for a questionnaire or interview study, which may include questions of a personal or distressing nature, ethics committee members will need to scrutinise the questionnaires with the same care they routinely give to participant information sheets. Even when the questionnaire seems incidental to the main study, copies must always be submitted to the ethics committee for scrutiny, as it is not unknown for such questionnaires to cause more ethical problems than the study itself.

Finally, to avoid causing distress to relatives, every effort should be made to ensure that the intended recipient is still alive before posting out the introductory letter and questionnaire to them.

Questionnaire studies are clearly by no means as innocuous as they may seem at first glance.

15

Epidemiological studies

Epidemiological studies have greatly improved the health of the population over the years. It has helped to clarify our understanding of the dangers to health, such as diseases due to drinking polluted water and smoking cigarettes. Some of this knowledge has led to changes in behaviour and to improved health. Examples are attitudes to: hygiene in food preparation; smoking, diet and exercise in relation to heart disease; and the wearing of seat belts to reduce the risk of death and serious injury from road traffic accidents.

Many epidemiological studies are based mainly on observation with no intervention more invasive than asking routine questions, reviewing case notes, or standard medical examinations. There are, however, other epidemiological studies where the questions can be more intrusive, like asking people about their drug injecting behaviour, when the maintenance of confidentiality assumes great importance. Some epidemiological studies may involve blood sampling and storage and physiological or psychological tests.

Types of epidemiological study

Retrospective case-controlled studies

Retrospective studies start with the disease and compare the history of exposure to, for instance cigarette smoke, in patients who have the illness with the exposure of people of similar age, sex and background who do not. This approach leads to observations that patients with certain forms of cancer are more likely to have been heavy smokers than matched controls, suggesting that smoking may be a factor in the development of the disease.

Prospective studies

Prospective studies (sometime known as cohort or longitudinal studies) take a different approach. They may look at individuals exposed to suspected risk factors, such as X-rays or industrial chemicals, and then follow them up for a number of years to see how many subsequently develop a disease, which it is suspected may be related to exposure to that agent. Alternatively, prospective studies may look at protective factors such as regular exercise or a healthy diet, following up individuals who have taken these on board, to determine whether or not in the long-term, they have a lower incidence of cardiovascular disease.

The application of information technology to large data sets has greatly expanded the capacity of epidemiological studies, enabling large numbers of people to be tracked over long periods of time.

Nutrition, an example of the ethical complexities of a typical national survey

A familiar kind of epidemiological study is the nutrition questionnaire designed to obtain more information about the diet of the population and to relate this to its past, present or future health. As was discussed in the previous chapter, many of these are done anonymously and raise few ethical issues. There are, however, more complex epidemiological studies that tend to raise a whole range of ethical issues that need to be addressed before the proposal can go ahead. To identify some of these issues, let us consider the example of a national survey of nutrition.

The overall aim of the study is to find out what people are eating these days, to establish the extent to which it is adequately nutritious and varied and to relate it to characteristics such as their age, sex, height and weight. It also aims to monitor over the years the extent to which the dietary targets set by the government are being met and to help develop strategies to help to achieve these targets.

What procedures will participants be exposed to?

In order to obtain the desired information, various methods will need to be used.

Diet – to derive nutrient intakes

To obtain detailed information on diet, participants will be asked to record everything they eat and drink for a number of consecutive days.

Ethical issues

Unlikely to raise any, except for confidentiality. Although most people do not mind others knowing what they eat, persons of certain religious groups (or nutrition experts) might be reluctant to reveal eating things they shouldn't unless assured that strict confidentiality will be maintained.

Urine – to estimate sodium intake

As reliable estimates of sodium cannot be obtained from dietary records, volunteers will provide a urine sample.

Ethical issues

Although the procedure itself does not appear to raise any ethical issues, problems may arise if there is a possibility of tests revealing abnormalities of relevance to patients. If this is a possibility, participants should be told beforehand how the situation would be handled.

Fasting blood sample – to provide indices of nutritional status
The blood sample is required for a variety of biochemical and hae-matological tests that will measure nutritional status – vitamins, minerals and fat levels – and the risk of nutrient deficiency.

Ethical issues
Participants should be told before giving consent for the blood test if it is intended to inform them of any test results found to be significantly outside the normal range, or to report such results to their family doctor. If it is intended to store blood samples, the purpose for which they will later be used should be stated. The patients should be contacted again and informed consent obtained before the samples are used for a purpose different from the original study.

Assessment of physical activity
This will involve completion of a physical activity diary and a questionnaire over a period of a week or so. A subsample of participants may have an assessment of physical activity made by an electronic monitor that they will wear.

Ethical issues
As it is not intended that their physical activity should change as a result of the study, there are no major ethical issues involved.

Physical measurements and blood pressure measurement and reporting
Blood pressure will be measured.

Ethical issues
The participants will need to agree to their family doctor being informed of the result if it is abnormal.

Oral health examination
An oral health examination will take place to examine the health of the teeth and gums.

Ethical issues
Participants will need to be told what the examination involves.

Flagging on a government or local register for follow-up contact
It may be desired in years to come to contact patients again in order
to see if their future health experience is related to their diet.

When informed consent must be obtained

This kind of epidemiological study clearly raises several concerns in relation to consent. The World Health Organization (WHO)
takes the view that informed consent must *usually* be sought from
participants in epidemiological studies (CIOMS/WHO 1991, s.11).

We have already established the wisdom of obtaining explicit
written consent for the following activities:

- Additional blood sample donation for tests of relevance to
  participants.
- Storage of spare blood samples, and again if they are subsequently
  to be used for a purpose different from the original.
- Provision of information to the participant's family doctor of the
  results of any tests found to have potential clinical significance.

To this list I would suggest adding:

- Flagging on a government or local register, which gives the
  researchers access to the participant following changes of address.

In obtaining consent, investigators must always emphasise to
potential subjects that participation in the survey is entirely voluntary and that they can withdraw at any time without giving a
reason. They must provide a full explanation of the nature and
purpose of the study and procedures involved. Participants should
be given a contact number to call if they have any queries about the
survey.

If children are included in the survey, information leaflets suitable for both young persons and their parents or guardians should be provided. The procedures used to obtain consent must adhere to strict ethical guidelines such as those published by the British Paediatric Association (1992). Issues associated with obtaining informed consent in children are discussed in more detail in Chapter 12.

With the participants' permission, it would be courteous to inform their family doctor by letter that they have agreed to participate in the study to enable the doctor to respond appropriately to any subsequent enquiry or incident. Participants must be given adequate time to consider and discuss the implication of the study with the investigator, friends and relatives or their family doctor.

Any young person who refuses or resists must have their wishes respected, regardless of any permission given by the parent or guardian. In a complex study such as the above, it may be appropriate to seek consent at each stage, allowing for co-operation with only some aspects of the study, so that children who wish to complete the dietary questionnaire without having the blood test may do so if they wish.

Incentives or rewards

No incentive or reward should be offered to participants for participation in any of the procedures listed above that require written consent. A small token of appreciation, probably in the form of a gift voucher, could be given to those who complete a part of the study that does not necessarily require written consent, such as a seven-day dietary record. Interviewers must make it clear to the participants that receipt of this token is *not* conditional on co-operation with any other aspect of the survey.

Contact numbers

The participants (or their parents/guardians) should be given a contact address and telephone number (preferably a free phone or evening off peak) for any queries.

Psychological tests

Epidemiologists whose questionnaires include intrusive questions of a psychological nature are referred to Chapter 14 for further discussion.

Epidemiological studies which may not require informed consent

An investigator who proposes *not* to seek informed consent must explain to the ethics committee how the study could be ethical in its absence (CIOMS/WHO 1991, s.2).

Non-intrusive questionnaire studies

In straightforward epidemiological studies, like the issuing of questionnaires to the general public about their dietary habits, the fact that they return the questionnaire may be taken as implied consent to be included in the study. If, however, an identifiable group, as for example, employees of the researcher is being asked to respond to a questionnaire, informed consent should be obtained. They will need to be assured that participation is entirely voluntary and that failure to participate will not affect their employment prospects.

The examination of medical records

Many epidemiological studies involve no more than the examination of medical records. This raises the question, discussed at length in Chapter 7, of whether patients need to be approached for their consent before researchers can look at their medical records.

Arguments against obtaining informed consent are that: (a) in large scale surveys involving computerised records, it may be impracticable to contact everyone involved to ask their permission; (b) informing subjects of their participation may change the behaviour that it is proposed to measure; and (c) people may be made needlessly anxious about why they have been selected to take part in research aimed at detecting the incidence of a serious illness. In agreeing to complete a simple questionnaire on their eating or smoking habits, do people really want to be told that following their death their medical records will be examined to see if the cause can be related to their replies to the questionnaire? Many people would not welcome such a vivid reminder of their mortality.

Confidentiality of data

When the study simply involves access to medical records, the main ethical issue is that of confidentiality. Provided that the investigator can provide evidence that confidentiality will be maintained, the ethics committee may agree that the researcher can proceed without contacting patients (Royal College of Physicians 1996, s.8.20–8.24). All surveys must be carried out in accordance with a strict code of confidentiality. No information must be released in a form in which it could be associated with an identifiable individual, without the individual's prior knowledge and consent. Storage of all data on computer must comply with the relevant legislation, which in the UK is the 1984 Data Protection Act (revised in 1998). The golden rule is that personal identifiers should be removed from the original data as soon as possible, so that patients are identified only by code. Once this has been done, the risk of individual breeches of confidentiality is minimal.

When a specific condition is being studied, and participants are to be contacted, great care must be taken when making the initial contact to avoid accidentally revealing to anyone opening a letter by mistake that the patient has the condition. This and other aspects of confidentiality are addressed in more detail in Chapter 7.

Confidentiality of groups

As well as its effect on individual participants, an epidemiological study can raise ethical problems if it results in a group or community suffering stigmatisation, prejudice, loss of prestige or self-esteem or economic loss, such as higher insurance premiums, as a result of taking part in the study. An example would be a study which found an excessively high consumption of alcohol among an ethnic minority in a particular area of the city, or a study that identified a high level of drug abuse funded by theft among young people on a certain housing estate, the results of which subsequently received wide press publicity. Researchers and medical research ethics committees need to be aware of these possibilities and to take steps to reduce the risk of them happening. Ideally in such studies, districts should be coded for the purposes of publication with their identity reserved for the professionals charged with tackling the social or medical problems identified by the study. In practice it may be necessary to point the finger at a district in order to bring help to it. In such cases the potential benefit must outweigh the likely harm.

In writing up a study for publication, investigators should realise that it may be read by journalists on the look-out for a good story and should therefore try to avoid saying anything that might be taken out of context.

Submission of proposals for epidemiological studies to the ethics committee

In view of the wide range of ethical issues that can be raised by seemingly innocuous epidemiological studies, investigators will need to be guided by their local medical research ethics committee as to whether the informed consent of participants is required for a particular study.

Genetic research – special ethical considerations

Before the advent of genetic screening it was recognised that certain conditions, such as haemophilia, ran in families and the broad pattern of inheritance could be worked out, but it could not be predicted with any degree of certainty which members of the family would get the disease until symptoms appeared. Today, once a genetic mutation associated with an inherited condition has been identified and screening methods devised, it is often possible to identify the actual individual who will suffer from the condition in advance of symptoms appearing, or the couple who are at high risk of bearing a child suffering from a particular disability. Testing may be done while the individual is still a fetus, shortly after birth or, in the case of conditions like Huntington's disease, which do not manifest themselves until later in life, at any stage during childhood or early adulthood. The ability to detect disorders in this way raises profound ethical issues that have been the subject of extensive debate (see 'Further reading').

In most kinds of research activity, the *risk* of harm to the participant has to be balanced against potential benefits. In contrast, in genetic screening it is often a case of balancing *actual* harm against potential benefits as most genetic research, unless done anonymously, causes anxiety and distress, especially to those participants who test positive, without necessarily bringing them personally any benefit.

This chapter focuses on the ethical regulation of the early stages of research into genetic diseases rather than the ethics of established screening programmes. This is characterised by an even greater level of uncertainty than surrounds established programmes. Great care has to be taken not to cause participants distress by introducing the possibility that they may be a carrier of a serious illness, only to discover later that the hypothesis was incorrect. Research may identify a mutation or gene variant which predisposes to a condition, only for the decision to be made that as there is no immediate prospect of prevention or treatment for those carrying it further screening would be inappropriate. As a result, participants may be left with distressing information about themselves, which is of no benefit to anyone.

With some types of inherited disease, a person who inherits two defective genes, one from the mother and one from the father will, as is the case with cystic fibrosis, the haemoglobinopathies and Tay–Sachs disease, almost certainly develop the disease, while with the autosomal dominant condition, Huntington's disease, only one defective gene is required. But such conditions are the exception rather than the rule. They were among the first to be researched and developed into screening programmes because they stood out as inherited conditions. More commonly, the relative influence of genes and environment is less clear cut, with inheritance of particular variants of a gene conferring an increased susceptibility to the condition in response to certain environmental factors. An increased tendency to lung cancer, for instance, may only manifest itself if the carrier of the gene conferring susceptibility is exposed to cigarette smoke. It is this kind of research which now forms the majority of applications to ethics committees.

In many established screening programmes, because of the relatively straight forward cause and effect of the mutations involved, geneticists are able to estimate with some degree of accuracy what proportion of family members are likely to have the mutation and the risk of developing the illness in later life or of passing it onto their children (although there are still likely to be uncertainties). With many of the conditions that are the object of current interest, it will take many years of painstaking research before a realistic assessment of risks and the possibility of successful interventions can be made, with what to tell participants creating an enormous dilemma for researchers at each stage of the process.

The following discussion will focus mainly on the initial research aimed at determining whether a condition has an inherited component and at identifying the genes implicated. There is a surprising lack of established ethical guidelines dealing with these early stages of genetic research. The following observations on the ethical issues involved and the need for caution at each stage of the process are therefore presented in an effort to stimulate further discussion.

Informed consent for genetic testing

Informed consent for participation in any kind of medical research where new information about the participant's health is to be generated is essential (CIOMS/WHO 1993, g.3; Royal College of Physicians 1996, s.73.1–74.9), and nowhere more so than in genetic testing, owing to the implications of a positive finding, both for the subjects themselves and for family members.

Researchers may be tempted to carry out genetic tests without consent on spare blood samples taken from patients for other reasons or on archived tissue. As more and more mutations and genetic variants creating susceptibility to particular diseases are identified, routine screening of everyone with cancer and heart disease and other conditions is fast becoming a reality. As this may be done by biomedical scientists with little experience of patients and their requirements, the need therefore for medical supervision is essential (World Medical Association 1996).

The temptation also exists to screen blood samples taken from well people, such as the extensive collections generated by screening for Down's syndrome, to determine the incidence of specific mutations in the general population. Only when done completely anonymously (Chapter 13) with no possibility of the results being traced back to the participant and when there are no ethical issues, is this acceptable. If anonymity cannot be guaranteed or there are ethical issues involved, such as prenatal screening which might prevent some participants from wishing to donate blood, informed consent is essential. If a stored sample is to be used for future tests, new consent must be obtained if the implications for the person at risk and their relatives resulting from the new research are significantly different from the original tests. This means that if it is intended to use blood taken for clinical purposes for genetic analysis, the patient's consent must be obtained first. If patients give explicit consent for their blood to be stored and retested as new DNA tests are developed, so long as the implications of a positive test for the patients and their relatives are the same as with the original test, it is not necessary to re-contact patients to obtain fresh consent. If, however, re-use of stored blood relates to genetic testing for different conditions, fresh consent must be obtained.

As part of the informed consent procedure, participants must be told: (a) exactly what the blood will be used for; (b) the implications of an abnormal finding for themselves and their relatives; (c), if an abnormality were found, whether they themselves or their family doctor would be informed; (d) the reliability of the test results; (e) plans for future use of the blood/tissue sample; (f) arrangements for confidentiality; and (g) the availability of counselling. Where a serious condition is involved the researcher should make it clear whether there are any circumstances in which there would be a moral obligation to contact relatives without the original patient's permission because of potential dangers to the relatives' health.

In the early stages of a new line of genetic research where the meaning and accuracy of results are yet uncertain, the researcher should normally make it clear to participants at the outset that neither they nor their family doctor will be informed of the results. They should be told that, if and when it is established that the condition is genetically determined and a reliable test developed, they can then be offered the opportunity to be re-tested if they wish.

When family doctors are informed of the results of genetic

testing of their patients, it is important to provide them with some guidance in the interpretation of the results, as the pace of developments in molecular biology is such that, unless the doctor has a special interest in the disorder, they may well not be completely up-to-date with the current state of genetic research in the area.

Aims of genetic research

Genetic research typically has one or more of the following aims:

- ► To determine whether a particular disease or susceptibility to it is inherited.
- ► To identify the gene or genes responsible.
- ► To work out what proportion of cases of the disease are the result of the defective gene. Can it also occur in patients who do not have the defective gene?
- ► To determine what proportion of people with the defective gene will go on to develop the genetic disorder later in life, and if not everyone does, the reasons why some do and some do not.
- ► To discover ways of preventing and treating the illness resulting from the genetic disorder or tendency to disease.
- ► To develop tests for the defective gene in the fetus to facilitate prenatal screening.
- ► To develop laboratory testing for the defective gene so that the test can be offered to all those who want it.
- ► To develop methods of gene therapy.

Although, for simplicity, I have referred to a 'defective gene', many genetic studies involve normal variants of a gene that are widely distributed in the population, but which may, under certain conditions, confer increased susceptibility to an illness or affect the likely outcome of the illness. The genetic defect may be identified directly by DNA analysis or indirectly, as traditionally with phenylketonuria, by observing its biochemical consequences.

If all of the above aims are to be achieved, it will be necessary at some point not only to identify and contact patients with the condition, but also to contact their relatives. This raises a host of ethical issues.

Identifying and approaching a patient with a known condition

Even when patients already know that they have a serious condition, contacting them with the proposition of investigating whether it has a genetic basis is always difficult in view of the profound implications this may have for themselves and their relatives and any decisions about having children.

Let us remind ourselves of some of the problems likely to be created for participants on learning that there is a strong genetic basis for their condition.

► If the condition is serious, it may be felt that they have a duty to tell their relatives so that they may also be tested, even though they would prefer that their condition remained confidential.

► Blame from a partner, or self-guilt, that they have passed on a disabling condition to their children.

► Should their spouse be tested to see if they have the same mutation which would result in a high probability of any children being affected?

► Should they decide not to have any (more) children?

► Alternatively should they go ahead and risk bearing a disabled child, or one who may develop the condition in later life?

► Should they abort a fetus which prenatal testing reveals is affected?

► Is the disability serious enough, or the results of the test reliable enough to justify abortion. Could they be aborting a normal child or one who would not be too seriously affected despite possessing the mutation, or be offending against their moral or religious beliefs?

In view of the extensive television coverage given to genetic diseases, it is likely that most people in developed countries with a long- standing illness will have wondered at some time or another if it might be partially inherited, especially if they have a relative who is similarly affected. An approach from a professional will, however, convert this vague curiosity into a serious concern.

A tactful approach is therefore essential. While doctors are trained to inspire the confidence of their patients, in the early stages of genetic research, full expression of the doubts and uncertainties that exist is eminently preferable. 'We would like to conduct research to determine whether there might be an inherited component to your illness which makes some people more likely to contract it than others in response to certain, presently unknown, environmental conditions,' is vastly preferable to a more confident approach that implies that the illness definitely is inherited and that it is simply a case of finding out if the patient has the inherited form which can be passed on to their offspring.

If the researcher is the patient's consultant or family doctor, the initial contact should present less of a problem as regards confidentiality. When, however, a researcher intends to contact patients of another doctor, identified from a Cancer Registration Database or other hospital records with a view to asking them if they wish to contribute to the project, the situation becomes more complex.

The first requirement is to be certain that all of the patients are fully aware that they have the disease. Not all patients will be aware of their diagnosis and a researcher revealing for the first time that patients have a cancer that they had not been told about will cause considerable distress. As a precaution, therefore, the approach should normally be made only with the agreement of the patient's family doctor and/or consultant who should ask their patient if they wish their name to be passed onto the researcher. This does not mean, however, that the family doctor necessarily has a right to know the outcome of the tests. Once a suspect gene has been identified in patients suffering from the condition, researchers may see contact with relatives as the next stage.

Implications for those not previously aware of a risk to their health

What sets genetic research apart from most other areas of research is the impact that it can have on persons other than the patient. It involves contacting people who are well, not as healthy controls, but to inform them that they or their relatives may be at risk of serious illness. Below is a list of some of the possible effects of contact.

- ► People may be devastated by the revelation that they may be at high risk of developing a serious condition in later life, or of being carriers of a serious condition which they may pass onto their children.
- ► The risk, from for example a gene that results in a higher risk of heart disease, may be low, but a disproportionate amount of anxiety be caused by the knowledge of carrying it.
- ► If the test proves negative, the initial anxiety may be relieved, unless they know that the test sometimes gives false negatives.
- ► Should the test prove positive, they will then face all of the problems of the original patient listed above.
- ► What will be the effect on an individual's insurance policies and employment prospects. Will insurers and employers find out, or have to be told?

The above are some of the problems necessarily faced by participants in *established* screening programmes. It will often be difficult, however, to justify generating these anxieties in a research project of uncertain outcome.

Should relatives be sought?

Relatives must not be contacted unless it is absolutely essential for the present stage of the research, especially if it concerns a serious late onset disease for which there is no effective treatment (Harper 1993). In early studies, where it is not known for certain whether the condition is inherited, preliminary information could be obtained by asking the sufferer to provide details of illnesses from which relatives, both living and dead, have suffered. In this case it would be the relative's confidential medical information that was being revealed without their consent, although as this was being done freely by a patient (a not unusual situation in a medical practice), there would not be a professional breach of confidentiality and so long as the information was kept strictly confidential by the researcher and not passed on to anyone else.

Before extending the research to relatives, the researcher should explore whether there is any work that should be done first to confirm the relationship between the mutation and the illness in known cases. In view of the serious implications of contacting relatives, every effort should be made to ensure that the required information could not be obtained in some other way.

The initial approach should be made by the researcher

Once patients agree that their relatives should be informed, the initial approach should normally be made by the researcher, rather than by the patients. The researcher is in a much better position to state what, if any, the increased risk of developing the condition might be, to put the risk into context and to offer advise and arrange for counselling. If the original patient insists on making the initial approach, as is often the case with serious conditions like breast and ovarian cancer, the researcher should provide an information leaflet for her to give to her relatives explaining the test and its implications, with a contact number for obtaining further information.

Avoid causing undue alarm

Once it has been agreed by the ethics committee that the stage and importance of the research justifies contacting relatives of the original patient, the next step is to determine how best to make the initial contact in view of the risk of alarming them by implying that they are at high risk of developing a serious illness.

Imagine a letter dropping through your letterbox, out of the blue, inviting you to participate in a research project. One of your relatives has a form of cancer which you always imagined they had contracted by chance, but now the researchers announce their belief that it may run in families and want to study you to help find out. What would your reaction be? With relatives, the vague approach advocated for the patient with the condition may not work. Even though the researchers stated that 'in *some* cases it *may* run in families' would you think they were just playing down the risk and that your days were numbered? If it were a disease for which there was no satisfactory treatment, perhaps you would rather have continued to live in blissful ignorance?

Researchers must take into account the fact that individual reactions vary considerably. While some people, for example smokers, seem to take a greatly increased risk of contracting a serious illness in their stride, others may become obsessed with the prospect and spend every waking moment for years to come on the lookout for symptoms. One approach might be to gain the help of the patient's family doctor, who will probably know the patient personally (though not necessarily, as not everyone visits their doctor regularly). Unfortunately, this would reveal that the patient was at risk before even agreeing to be tested, which is contrary to the rule that genetic testing should not be done without the patient's informed consent.

In genetic studies, considerable thought has to be given to the initial approach to patients' relatives and the potential, long-term psychological harm that an insensitive approach could cause.

Random population screening and screening of controls

While less likely to generate the initial alarm and anxiety of a personal approach to a relative, population screening for a potentially harmful mutation clearly has profound implications for those who test positive and, unless done anonymously, participants must be fully informed of the implications of a positive test. In view of the difficulties, would it be preferable not to contact patients at all? While anonymous testing for serious conditions has a well known precedent in the testing of blood samples during pregnancy for HIV, to gain preliminary figures of incidence, it should not be encouraged simply to avoid the problems associated with dealing with patients if the results would be of real value to them or their relatives. In the early stages of genetic research, anonymous testing to assess the frequency of the mutation in the general population may be an acceptable approach.

The problem of explaining risks

The risk of possessing the mutation

If it is considered necessary and acceptable to approach relatives for genetic testing, the chance of them harbouring the suspect gene and of contracting the disease should be clearly explained, as far as is known, in every day terms. If, as is often the case, it is not known, this should be openly stated. If it is not known, this could well be because the risk is comparatively low, and few families with multiple affected members have been identified. The risk will depend on the way in which the disease is inherited. At one extreme it may be a virtual certainty, at the other only slightly higher than that of the general population. In cases where the research ultimately shows that the disease is not inherited, any increased risk may be because other members of the family smoke or engage in other dangerous activities and have nothing to do with genetic susceptibility.

Researchers may sometimes be tempted to over emphasise the potential risk in an effort to attract interest in and funding for their research proposal. While the ethics of doing so in a research grant application are outside the scope of this guide, this enthusiasm must not be allowed to spill over into the patient information sheet.

The risk of illness for a person possessing the mutation

The degree of 'increased risk' conferred by the mutation or gene variant must be specified, if known. Patient information sheets that speak of an 'increased risk' frequently fail to specify that risk, leaving participants to imagine the worst when the increased risk may turn out to be marginal or non-existent, similar perhaps to that involved in travelling to work rather than staying at home. It is irresponsible to tell people that if they carry a certain mutation they have an increased risk of heart disease or some other condition without specifying the risk if known.

Consideration also has to be given to the possibility that some genetic variations, while resulting in an increased risk of one disease may help to confer protection against another. A well-known example of this phenomenon is the mutation in the hae-moglobin gene that increases the risk of sickle cell anaemia whilst protecting the affected individual against malaria in countries where malaria is endemic.

Risks are relative

It should also be explained to patients that risks are relative. An individual might well be alarmed to be told that they were ten times more likely to get a certain kind of skin cancer because of their genetic makeup than the general population. This statement could easily apply to any white skinned person living in an area with a mainly black skinned population, while the same person living in a mainly white area would have a risk no greater than that of the general population.

The actual risk will also depend on how common the illness is. For a man to be told that he is four times more likely to get breast cancer than other men should not cause him any great concern as the incidence in men is so low that, even with the increased risk, the chances of him contracting it are negligible. For a woman, the same information will cause far greater concern as the average risk in women is already so much higher. The fact that so many people in the UK play the National Lottery emphasises the extent to which the concept of probabilities can get distorted. If you believe that you have a chance of winning the lottery jackpot with odds of less than one in ten million then the chance of getting a particular kind of cancer when you are told that the odds are one in a hundred may seem like a certainty.

Ensure that adequate counselling is available

Counselling, both by a geneticist who can give a clear indication of the risk and potential medical consequences for patients and their relatives, born and unborn, and by a counsellor trained in dealing with emotional and psychological problems, should always be available for patients introduced to the possibility that they may be at significantly greater risk of a serious condition because of the way it is inherited. As only relatively small numbers of people are involved in most research projects, it should be possible to offer a higher level of support and advice than in established programmes. Even so, the cost implications are likely to be considerable, and whenever possible should be built into the initial funding proposals.

It should not be assumed, however, that counselling, no matter how expert the counsellor, will necessarily be of any benefit once the seeds of despair are sown. In the early stages of the development of a screening test for a particular disorder, counsellors are often at a considerable disadvantage, as basic information on the risks of transmission may not yet be available to them.

In addition to scrutinising the literature on the subject, researchers should themselves undergo a mock counselling session based on the possible outcomes of their research, to give themselves greater personal insight into the likely reaction of patients on learning that they possess a harmful mutation.

If only a small proportion, say one in several hundred, of the individuals tested are likely to carry the mutation, as is usually the case when the general population is screened for a mutation (the familiar cystic fibrosis gene has an exceptionally high incidence of around 1 in 25 of the population), detailed counselling for all may be impractical and researchers may prefer to reserve it for those who test positive. The implications of a positive finding must, however, be carefully explained during the informed consent procedure and participants informed in the patient information sheet of the detailed counselling arrangements that will be available for those who test positive.

Each study will have to be considered on its merits by the ethics committee, a major influencing factor being the severity of the condition. If possession of the mutation has dire consequences for anyone testing positive, it may be desirable, despite the problems, to offer counselling to *all* participants before they agree to the test.

Advantages and disadvantages of early detection

Early detection of serious late onset diseases with no immediate prospect of a treatment

A particular problem arises in the case of research into serious conditions that, like Huntington's disease, do not appear until later in life. This raises the question of whether people really want to be informed now that they are destined to suffer a serious illness in 20 years time.

The answer will be influenced by whether there is any satisfactory treatment available. If not, can it be ethical to tell people that they are likely to die of a disease in 20 years time if there is absolutely nothing that can be done to reduce the risk? The situation becomes yet more complex when we realise that their children and relatives may also be affected and that such knowledge may be necessary to enable them to make sound reproductive decisions.

When early detection may facilitate attempts at prevention

In regard to the genetic testing of children, the British Paediatric Association (1992, p.8) warns: 'with research into serious disorders which present in adult life, presymptomatic diagnosis in a child, while it may be beneficial, may also have very harmful effects, and may affect the child's opportunities and freedom of choice'.

Parents and adoption agencies frequently request paediatricians to carry out genetic testing to predict diseases that occur later in life, but should they? The same issues arise as with genetic testing for late onset diseases in young adults with the additional problem that the children are too young to give properly informed consent themselves. There is no consensus view on this. My own view is that testing of this type in young children is only acceptable when symptoms of the condition normally occur in childhood, or when there is a useful treatment that can be offered, such as a special diet or medication. To test a six-year-old for a condition known as polyposis coli, in which there is a high risk of cancer of the colon, might therefore be acceptable, if there is a family history, as regular surveillance could pick up early cancers and improve outcome.

At the other extreme, if the adult disease is currently untreatable, as is the case with Huntington's disease, genetic testing should *not* be done in a young child. Formal genetic testing should wait until the child specifically requests the test and is capable of understanding the consequences sufficiently to give informed consent. To test a healthy six-year-old for Huntington's disease because of a family history is unacceptable as nothing could be done to prevent the condition if the test should prove positive, and the child's early years of life would be irretrievably blighted. The same principle applies to any other condition for which there is no prospect of treatment. The situation is, however, complicated by the fact that the reality usually lies somewhere in between.

If there were an effective means of prevention and/or effective treatment, it is a reasonable assumption that most people would want to be told that they were at increased risk of an illness no matter how potentially serious. The typical situation with inherited late onset diseases, however, is that although there are potential treatments that could be used and may prove beneficial, until proper clinical trials are conducted, no one can say for certain if they will be. Early diagnosis is often essential if patients are to be entered into such trials. Take the example of familial hypercholesterolaemia, a genetic disorder that increases levels of cholesterol in the bloodstream. The affected person is therefore at increased risk of heart disease. It is a reasonable proposition that the introduction of a low fat diet early in life and treatment with drugs that lower blood cholesterol levels may reduce the risk of premature heart disease, but this treatment cannot be implemented until the condition is diagnosed, and the patient informed. It can be argued that diagnosis in childhood is essential in order to develop an effective treatment for the condition. With this and other comparable conditions the acceptability or otherwise of testing in the young depends on the strength of the scientific evidence that the interventions are likely to be of benefit. Also to be taken into account are the results of any previous work on compliance with treatment in the age group concerned. If it is extremely low, it may not be worthwhile diagnosing the condition so early.

The right of participants *not* to know should be respected

Many doctors feel it their duty to tell patients the truth no matter how upsetting it may be to patients initially, as they believe the knowledge may help them 'to make informed choices about their lives'. As so often in life, there are double standards. We all have colleagues who drive too fast and therefore have a greatly increased risk of killing themselves or, worse still, someone else, but do we feel it our duty to point this out to them and offer them counselling? Ironically, in this case counselling, if successful, could eliminate the excess risk.

The truth of the matter is that not everyone willing to participate in a genetic study to help further the advance of knowledge will wish to know the results of their test. They must be given the option not to know and this wish respected.

Confidentiality in genetic studies

Confidentiality is of the utmost importance in all aspects of genetic research. If confidential information about a participant's susceptibility to a serious genetic condition is revealed, there is the possibility of stigmatisation in the search for a job or insurance. When the information may be of value to participants or their relatives, the risks of a breach of confidentiality may be worth taking. When, however, the information is likely to result in harm to participants, it may not be. The search for genetic factors associated with 'intelligence' if it led to widespread genetic testing by educational establishments and employers could lead to stigmatisation of individuals on a massive scale, and is an area of research where international regulation is urgently required.

It should be understood that a researcher does not have the automatic right to know about the genetic makeup of an individual, but must obtain consent before performing genetic testing. It has to be recognised, however, that in examining a family tree, information may be deduced by the researcher about the genetic constitution of people who have never been screened. In examining family trees with a patient, care must be taken not to reveal confidential information about other members of the family.

The patient's permission must be obtained first

If contact is considered essential, it must be remembered that relatives should not normally be approached without the permission of the patient, as to do so might well result in confidential medical information being revealed to relatives who were not previously aware of it. Seriously ill parents, for example, may wish to conceal the true nature of their illness from their children for as long as possible. In established screening programmes, there is debate about whether the relatives' right to know their genetic status, particularly if they are at risk of a serious late onset disease or of having a severely disabled child, should override the right to confidentiality of the index case who does not wish the condition to be disclosed to family members (Nuffield Council on Bioethics 1993, s.55–5.7).

To give a concrete example, a study to establish what proportion of women under the age of 30 with ovarian cancer have a defective gene which strongly predisposes to this condition has ethical implications even if done anonymously. This is because it raises the question of whether, when a patient is found to have the defective gene, it is right to keep the information from herself and from her relatives. If her relatives knew, it might give them the opportunity to be tested for the gene too, so that anyone who proved positive could be offered a prophylactic oophorectomy or regular screening to catch the disease at an early stage, although it is still to be established whether such early intervention really does save lives.

In the early stages of a new line of genetic research, when the meaning and accuracy of results is uncertain, there is rarely the same imperative to override the duty of confidentiality to the original patient to contact at-risk relatives.

In terms of confidentiality, a distinction may be drawn between genetic tests performed during a research project and those performed during an established screening programme. In view of the high degree of uncertainty surrounding the meaning of results obtained in preliminary research and in many cases the rate of false negatives and false positives, such research results should not normally be transmitted to a third party without first being anonymised. Under the terms of the UK Data Protection Act 1984 it is the duty of researchers to ensure that computerised data is accurate. If participants were harmed as a result of inaccurate data being transmitted to an employer or insurance company, they would be within their rights to sue the researcher concerned. When there is significant uncertainty regarding the meaning and accuracy of results, family members should not be contacted without the approval of the original patient, if at all.

In view of the potential impact of genetic information, not only on the patient immediately concerned, but also on family members, the strictest rules of confidentiality must apply when genetic data are entered onto a computerised database. The following advise is based on that given in Chapter 7 for databases of serious illness in general.

▶ The patient's permission must be obtained first. The researcher should provide a simple information sheet and consent form for patients to sign if they agree to be included on the register.

▶ The information must be anonymised before registration on the database (CIOMS/WHO 1991, g.26) by deleting names and addresses and dates of birth and by allocating a code number. Holding a simple list of names and addresses corresponding to the code numbers in a locked cupboard remote from the main register will enable the codes to be broken by the principal researcher if required.

▶ Confidentiality can be improved by omitting the name of the patient's family doctor or consultant from the file and referring to them too only by code number.

▶ The exclusion of confidential patient information is especially important if the computer is attached to a network.

There is concern among researchers that the media attention given to the potential interest of insurance companies in confidential genetic information could influence the willingness of patients to take part in valuable genetic research (Daniel 1997). The researcher must therefore be able to assure the participant that the data will be kept in a form in which neither an employer nor insurance company would be able to gain access.

Social stigmatisation

The unauthorised release of confidential information regarding individuals is not the only concern. Stigmatisation of ethnic or social groups may result if they are found to have an increased predisposition to a particular condition, whether medical or behavioural. Potentially one of the most serious scenarios would be if a particular ethnic or social group came to be stigmatised as a result of publicity following screening for genes associated with intelligence.

Where social stigmatisation could conceivably result from the publication of the results of genetic screening, I would recommend that the ethics committee, if approving the study, should do so only on condition that results identifying groups will not be reported without prior scrutiny by, and written approval of, the ethics committee and the researchers' employing institution.

It should not be supposed, however, that genetic studies are exempt from the basic principles of the Declaration of Helsinki (World Medical Association 1996) that,

> Biomedical research involving human subjects cannot legitimately be carried out unless the importance of the objective is in proportion to the inherent risk to the subject. (Article I 4.)

And

> Every biomedical research project involving human subjects should be preceded by careful assessment of predictable risks in comparison with foreseeable benefits to the subject and others (Article I.5.)

Unless the researcher can provide convincing evidence that the potential benefits of such research override the potential risks, the ethics committee has a duty not to allow it to go ahead. The satisfying of academic curiosity does not in itself constitute a benefit.

Development of new methods of prenatal diagnosis

The ability to detect in the fetus the genetic defects that give rise to conditions such as Down's syndrome or cystic fibrosis, raises important ethical issues for parents who are offered the test. But what are the issues facing an individual being invited to participate in a study which may in the long-term lead to the development of a new method of prenatal diagnosis or the ability to screen for other conditions?

To illustrate some of the ethical issues that arise from research aimed at expanding the potential of prenatal diagnosis, let us consider the following scenario. The methods currently available for identifying genetic problems in the child prior to birth involve amniocentesis and chorionic villus sampling. Unfortunately both techniques, especially the latter, can result in miscarriage, infection and occasionally malformations. The ability to conduct prenatal diagnosis on the small number of fetal cells that get into the mothers blood during pregnancy, obtained from a blood sample taken from the mother's arm early in pregnancy would eliminate the possibility of miscarriage or damage to the fetus. If the study succeeded in establishing the feasibility of obtaining sufficient fetal cells from the mother's blood for genetic testing, at least three important consequences would ensue.

► The new method would eventually replace amniocentesis and chorionic villus sampling with their risks of miscarriage. This is an advance in safety that many people would regard as, *in itself*, ethically sound.

► The increase in safety may encourage more women to undergo these tests. This would increase the number of positive results, and consequently the moral dilemma facing those found to be positive, and possibly the number of abortions.

▶ With research material now so readily available, the development of tests for a wider range of genetic abnormalities would be speeded up, with each one creating yet more major ethical issues.

Ultimate responsibility for the ethical assessment of the proposal is likely to fall on the parents

Although individual members of a medical research ethics committee might abstain from the discussion, the likelihood is that most ethics committees would approve research aimed at developing a more effective method of prenatal diagnosis for a lethal or seriously disabling condition. This raises the question of for what conditions prenatal genetic testing should be allowed. With abortions being carried out daily for what at times may appear the most trivial of social reasons, there is every danger that such knowledge might be abused in the vain search for the 'perfect child'.

The British Medical Association (1993, s.4:9.2.1) takes the view that prenatal genetic testing should not be carried out for frivolous reasons to detect traits not associated with a disease condition. This obviates the possibility of requests for the abortion of fetuses that would give rise to people of, for example, higher or lower than average stature. I would also suggest that prenatal testing is only appropriate for conditions like glaucoma or psoriasis which do not normally result in severe lifelong disability or early death, if the purpose of early detection is to initiate treatment to limit the effect of the condition following birth. Prenatal testing for genetic factors associated with 'intelligence' should not be permitted.

While prenatal testing is currently limited by the risks associated with amniocentesis and chorionic villus sampling, the ability to isolate fetal cells from the maternal circulation may make prenatal testing for a variety of genetic conditions as convenient as adult testing. It is therefore important that researchers are aware of the need to obtain prior approval from their local medical ethics committee for each trait for which they wish to develop tests.

In studies that gain ethical approval, the ultimate decision whether or not to participate will be left with the parents. Women who are opposed to abortion may not wish to be involved in the development of techniques for obtaining information that might lead to other women being offered abortions. Neither may their partners. They might well be extremely distressed and angry if they were to find out that a routine blood sample had also been used for this purpose without their knowledge. As emphasised in the discussion in Chapter 13, spare tissue samples must never be used for ethically controversial purposes without first obtaining the written informed consent of the donors. A woman's decision may be influenced by the nature of the condition being studied. Some women would find prenatal testing for a condition that invariably results in the death of the infant within a month of birth more acceptable than testing for genetic mutations giving say an extra finger on the hands of an otherwise healthy baby.

It is vitally important that there should be no undue persuasion. It should be made easy to say 'No', preferably by means of a tick on a form, rather than having to suffer the embarrassment of a face-to-face refusal. This is particularly important in an obstetrics department that has come to take prenatal testing for granted.

To facilitate informed consent in regard to prenatal testing, the researcher must ensure that the participant is fully aware of all of the long-term implications of the research being proposed. The most preliminary of studies designed to determine whether or not a particular condition is genetically determined may ultimately lead to prenatal testing and the option of abortion. If this is a possibility, for consent to be valid, the potential outcome of the research should be stated in the participant information sheet. Prospective participants will need adequate time in which to make their decision, as it is important that they are not pressurised into doing something that they will later regret.

If the study involves cell or tissue culture, the researcher must not omit to tell the participants that, in order to obtain enough cells to work on, these cells will be grown in culture. Should a miscarriage occur, this might mean that the cultured cells were kept alive after the death of the baby, an idea that might distress some parents. Even the most basic of studies aimed at the prenatal diagnosis of genetic defects are an ethical minefield. The greatest of care must be taken in asking people to help in studies involving prenatal diagnosis to avoid encouraging them to do anything which might go against their moral or religious beliefs.

In an effort to ensure that consent is valid, the patient information sheet/consent form should include the additional information listed at the end of this chapter.

When the outcome of genetic research becomes normal clinical practice

In research studies, the possibility of patients discovering that they are genetically susceptible to a disease stems from the researcher's desire to determine if the disease has a genetic origin. Once the genetic basis of a condition is established and screening for it introduced, the fact that it runs in families will soon become general knowledge. Anyone with a relative with the condition will suspect that they themselves may also be at risk.

It is common knowledge that Huntington's disease and certain forms of breast and ovarian cancer are inherited, as a result of which relatives of affected persons frequently ask to undergo testing to see if they have inherited the gene. In contrast, others will not wish to know and decline the offer if approached.

The impact of genetic screening on an individual

To summarise some of the dilemmas raised by genetic testing by reference to the story of a young man who finds that he has a serious wasting disease – such as, myotonic dystrophy – inherited from his mother.

▶ Knowing that it is likely to affect his performance of the job in the future, should the young man inform his employer? If he applies for another job should he tell his prospective employer, knowing that this will almost certainly eliminate any chance of being shortlisted? Does his new employer have a right to obtain this knowledge from his family doctor as part of a pre-employment medical? Must he tell his insurance company who will then refuse to renew his policies or put up his premiums?

► Should he tell his sisters, so that they can get tested? Do they have a legal and/or moral right to know?

► One of his sisters gets tested and finds that she has the mutation. This means that although she is not likely to be seriously affected herself, there is a 50:50 chance that she has already passed it onto her young son.

► As there is a similar chance that if she has another son, she will pass it onto him, should she decide not to have any more children?

► Should the existing son be tested? If he were found to have the condition, the parents might become over protective and as there is no treatment for the condition nothing could be done. On the other hand, if they knew that he was going to be affected in a certain way physically, they could try and direct his education so that he entered a career where physical strength and precise co-ordination were not required. What should the family do? Should the child be allowed to make his own decision when he is old enough to decide?

Should I accept the test?

Below is a summary of the advantages and disadvantages of genetic testing as it applies to the individual in severe conditions such as Huntington's disease where possession of the defective gene results in a high risk of developing the illness.

Why you might want to know if you have the gene

► To enable you to plan your life.
► To help with the decision about marriage and having a family.

▶ Reassurance if you do not have the gene.

▶ To provide information of importance to your children.

▶ If you have the gene and it becomes possible to prevent the disease you can make use of the preventative measures.

▶ You may be the sort of person who wants to know as much as possible about yourself and your future and find it hard to live with uncertainty.

●●●●● **Why you might *not* want to know you have the gene**

▶ You may not be willing to change your plans regarding marriage and having a family whatever the test result.

▶ You prefer to live with uncertainty and to plan your life without knowing your genetic status.

▶ If you have the gene the information may limit your opportunities, for example in relation to career choices, life insurance and financial matters.

▶ You do not think you could cope with knowing that you had the gene and had a high risk of developing the disorder.

Doctors should remind their patients that if they do not take the test now, they are always free to change their mind and can take the test in the future if, for example, a treatment becomes available that can prevent the disease. On the other hand, once the test is done and they know the results there is no going back.

Many of the genetic tests currently under development will not, in the foreseeable future, be capable of revealing more than an increased susceptibility to a condition. It will not be possible to predict with any degree of accuracy, the severity, nor even whether the disease will manifest itself at all. With many late onset conditions, the infected fetus may have as many as 40 or 50 years of disease-free life before symptoms of the condition arise. An above average risk of a disabling condition arising in middle age could surely never justify considering the termination of an affected fetus, especially as medical advances might eventually improve the outcome.

Research involving genetic testing

● ● ● ● ● ● ● ● ● **Proposed guidelines**

▶ It must be accepted that a researcher does not have the automatic right to know about the genetic makeup of an individual.

▶ Informed, written consent must be obtained before genetic testing is first carried out on fresh, spare or archived blood or other tissue samples, even when this means re-contacting participants for consent several years after the sample was taken. This requirement can only be waived if the testing is done anonymously and if there are no ethical issues, such as prenatal testing, involved.

● ● ● ● ● ● ● ● ● **Contacting patients with a known disease to determine if it has a genetic basis**

▶ When the tests are designed to determine if there is a genetic basis to an illness, care must be taken before contacting patients to ensure that they are fully aware that they have the illness.

▶ A researcher not previously involved in the patient's care should obtain the agreement of the family doctor and/or consultant before making the initial approach.

▶ Prior consent from patients must, however, be obtained if it is intended to communicate any apparent abnormal findings to their family doctor, in view of the fact that such information may then become accessible to insurers or potential employers.

▶ If a sample is to be stored and used for future tests, new consent must be obtained if the implications for the person at risk and their relatives resulting from the new research are significantly different from the original test (e.g., if genetic testing is to be done on samples not taken for this purpose, or if a different illness is involved from that investigated by the original test).

▶ Consent for *unspecified* future use of stored blood/tissue is not acceptable.

▶ When a high degree of uncertainty exists surrounding the meaning and accuracy of results obtained in preliminary research, such results should not normally be communicated to the patient or to the family doctor, or placed in their case notes. They should not be transmitted to other research groups without first being anonymised. Once a standard screening test is developed, patients can be re-contacted and offered the opportunity of having a fresh blood sample taken if they wish.

Contacting relatives of the original patient

▶ Samples should not be obtained from family members at risk, unless this is strictly necessary for the research. This applies particularly if it concerns a serious disease for which there is no effective treatment and particularly if children are involved.

▶ If contact is considered essential, relatives should not normally be approached without the permission of the original patient.

▶ This rule may only be overridden with the approval of the ethics committee if serious damage to the health of relatives is likely if they are not informed. If the patient is deceased and the results are thought to be important for family members, the local medical ethics committee should be approached for advice.

▶ Once patients agree that their relatives should be informed, the initial approach should normally be made by the researcher, rather than by the patients.

▶ If patients, despite advice to the contrary, insist on making the first contact, a detailed information sheet should be provided, which would normally be part of the informed consent procedure, to give to their relatives, with a contact number for further information.

▶ The risks of possessing and suffering ill effects from the harmful gene should not be exaggerated in order to encourage the participation of relatives.

▶ Adequate counselling must be available for patients at high risk of serious illness or giving birth to a seriously disabled child both prior to screening and again if the test is positive.

▶ It is acceptable to test for late onset diseases in children under 16 only if there is strong scientific evidence that early intervention is likely to be of benefit and if a high level of compliance with the treatment is likely to be achieved.

► The strictest rules of confidentiality must be followed (page 119) if computerised case registers are to be developed by researchers for holding details of people who have particular inherited illnesses or genetic traits. Names and addresses must be physically separated from medical details (e.g., a paper list kept in a locked cabinet) with patients identified on the database only by code number.

► To ensure the involvement of someone with experience of working with patients, genetic screening carried out by students or non-clinical scientists should be done either under the supervision of a qualified medical practitioner or involve such a person as a co-researcher.

Population screening and controls

► If testing is not done anonymously, all participants in a study to determine the frequency of a mutation in the general population must give written informed consent prior to testing so that they are aware of the implications of a positive test for themselves and their relatives, and adequate counselling must be made available for those who test positive. As it must never be assumed that all members of a control group will test negative, informed consent for testing is again of great importance.

Prenatal genetic testing

► To reduce the risk of more abortions being carried out for seemingly trivial reasons, research into methods of prenatal testing for conditions that are not severely disabling should only be permitted if the clear aim is to initiate early treatment following birth.

► In research into techniques of prenatal testing it must always be made easy for women opposed to abortion to refuse to participate, preferably by ticking a 'No' box on a form rather than having to suffer the embarrassment of declining an offer from an enthusiastic researcher face-to-face.

Ethical approval

▷ All studies involving genetic screening must be approved by a medical research ethics committee prior to commencement even if performed anonymously on spare blood samples.

▷ As with all biomedical research, the committee must only approve the study if it is convinced that the importance of the objective is in proportion to the inherent risk to the subjects, whether the subjects are individuals or ethnic or social groups.

▷ All amendments to the original approved protocol must be approved by the committee prior to implementation.

Informed consent for genetic testing – additional items to be included on the participant information sheet

▷ State exactly what the blood or other tissue samples will be used for.

▷ Describe the implications of an abnormal finding for the original patient and their relatives.

▷ State what stage of development the research has reached and, consequently, how reliable the results are likely to be. State the chance of false positives or false negatives.

▷ Specify as far as is known the likelihood that the condition is genetically inherited.

▷ State whether:
(a) the participants themselves will be told the results of testing;
(b) their family doctor will be told;
(c) results will be recorded in their case notes.

▷ State whether their insurers or prospective employers will be able to gain access to this information?

▷ State if there is any likelihood that the researchers may wish in the future to contact relatives, and make it clear that their (the original patient's) permission would be requested prior to this.

▷ Make it clear if there are any circumstances in which relatives would be contacted without the patient's permission.

▷ Describe what arrangements for counselling are available both to the original patient and, if appropriate, their relatives, prior to testing and/or in the event of a positive result.

▶ State if cell or tissue culture might be involved.

▶ If there is any possibility of the commercial exploitation of a cell line derived from the participant, this should be stated and, if so, whether the permission of the participant would be sought first.

▶ Participants should be advised that stored blood will not be used for testing for any other illness or genetic trait which is not the subject of the present study without first obtaining their written permission.

▶ If applicable, state the risk of miscarriage caused by a prenatal diagnostic procedure.

▶ When the accuracy and meaning of the results is currently too uncertain to be communicated to participants, they should be asked whether, if and when a standard screening test is developed, they wish to be re-contacted and given the opportunity of taking the test.

▶ Patients must be asked if they agree to their blood samples being used in the future if appropriate new tests become available to further investigate the genetic basis of their illness.

▶ State that participants have a right *not* to know the results, and give them the option of recording on the consent form that they do not wish to be informed of them.

17

Gene therapy

What is gene therapy?

At its most straightforward, gene therapy means inserting a synthetic gene into the cells of a patient to replace a defective gene, which is resulting in a particular illness.

A gene is a sequence of deoxyribonucleic acid (DNA), which contains the instructions for making a particular protein. Humans have at least 50,000 different genes working together, although only about 10 per cent are used in any one type of cell. Inherited differences between individuals are due to differences in their genes. A defect in the structure of a particular gene may result in a defective protein being made. If the protein has an essential role in the body and can not function properly because of the defect, a specific illness, such as cystic fibrosis, may result.

Steps leading to gene therapy

Once it has been established that a particular condition is inherited, the development of gene therapy involves the following steps:

(1) The identification of the defective gene.
(2) The normal gene must be isolated and copies of it produced in large amounts.
(3) It must be incorporated into a delivery system, such as the fatty droplets known as liposomes, specially modified retroviruses, or plasmids.

(4) Using these delivery systems the gene must be inserted into the cells of the patient, preferably specifically into those cells where the gene is normally expressed (by 'expressed' is meant that it directs the production of a protein which performs an essential function).

(5) Once inside the cell, the synthetic gene must be able to direct the production of the required protein in much the same way as the normal gene would have done.

Getting normal genes into affected cells

Injecting a gene into a patient is not an effective way of getting it into their cells. The DNA has to be transported into the cell by means of some sort of carrier, usually a virus, a liposome or a plasmid.

Retroviruses

Viruses may be used in gene therapy to carry genes into cells. The retroviruses used for this purpose are generally of animal origin and are not ones known to cause diseases in humans. They are genetically engineered to make them safe so that they can transport a gene for gene therapy into human cells without causing disease.

Liposomes

These are specially formulated droplets of fat containing the manufactured gene that can fuse with cell membranes and allow the genes to enter the cell.

Plasmids

Plasmids are circular pieces of DNA usually obtained from bacteria that, in nature, transfer genes from one kind of bacteria to another. Genetically engineered plasmids are used in some gene therapy trials instead of viruses.

Regulation of gene therapy

The European Joint Statement on Gene Therapy

In 1988, the medical research councils of 11 western European nations, including the UK, produced a joint statement (Gene Therapy Advisory Committee 1995) which recommended that:

▶ Gene therapy should be limited to efforts to correct diseases or defects.

▶ It should be limited to body cells and that no attempt should be made at this stage to insert defective genes into sperm cells or embryos.

▶ Initial research should emphasise the development of safe methods of delivering a replacement gene.

▶ There is a need to agree national guidelines for good practice and to establish national bodies to oversee clinical trials.

The first protocol for a gene therapy experiment on humans was approved by the Recombinant DNA Advisory Committee of the US National Institutes of Health, in 1988. In the following year, the Advisory Committee published its guidelines: *Points to Consider in the Design and Submission of Human Somatic Cell Gene Therapy Protocols* (National Institutes of Health 1989).

Background to gene therapy regulation in the UK

In 1989, the UK government set up the Committee on the Ethics of Gene Therapy, under the chairmanship of Sir Cecil Clothier. Its task was to draw up ethical guidance for the medical profession on the treatment of genetic disorders in adults and children by genetic modification of human body cells. The Committee reported in 1992 (Clothier 1992).

The recommendations of the Clothier committee

A researcher contemplating research in gene therapy or a local research ethics committee likely to be given the task of reviewing a proposal for gene therapy, should refer to the original report (Clothier 1992). Among its main recommendations are:

- All attempts at gene therapy should be regarded, at least initially, as research, and not as ordinary medical practice. It should, therefore, be controlled by standards that are as high as those already applying to other medical research (s.4.2).
- In the present state of knowledge, gene therapy research should remain restricted to disorders that are life threatening or cause serious handicap and for which treatment is either unavailable or unsatisfactory (s.4.3).
- Every effort should be made to obtain consent which is as fully informed as current knowledge allows, with all patients so treated being made fully aware of the uncertainties (s.4.11).
- All gene therapy must be directed to alleviating disease in individuals and germ line therapy should not yet be permitted (s.5.1– 5.2).
- A new expert advisory body – a Gene Therapy Advisory Committee – should be set up, which would include experts who could assess the scientific merit, benefits and risks, the legal implications, and wider public concerns of all proposals for gene therapy research (s.6.2).
- All gene therapy research must be approved by the Gene Therapy Advisory Committee and by the appropriate local research ethics committee (s.6.3–6.4). Only after approval by *both* committees can patients be approached to participate.
- Gene therapy should be confined to a small number of centres whilst experience is gained (s.7.12).
- It was concluded that the ethical issues raised by gene therapy limited to body cells are similar to those raised in other kinds of medical research and that gene therapy raises no special ethical issues (s.4.23).

The Gene Therapy Advisory Committee established as a result of the recommendations held its first meeting at the end of 1993 .

Other bodies with responsibilities in gene therapy research

As well as the Gene Therapy Advisory Committee and the local medical research ethics committees, other bodies have interests and responsibilities in relation to gene therapy research. These include the Medicines Control Agency (MCA), which has responsibility for regulating the handling and preparation of medicinal products, and applications for their use in clinical trials. Any proposal to conduct gene therapy research in the UK should, therefore, also be notified to the MCA.

The system of review in the USA is similar in overall structure to that developed in the UK, including assessment by a specialist national advisory committee, local ethical consideration by institutional review boards, and licensing by the appropriate medicines authority.

Gene therapy in practice

In order to gain a feel for what gene therapy is capable of, a sample of the research proposals put before the Committee on the Ethics of Gene Therapy and then the Gene Therapy Advisory Committee (GTAC 1995) in its first year of operation will be discussed.

The replacement of defective genes by new ones
Cystic fibrosis

This is one of the most common inherited serious diseases in the UK, affecting nearly 7000 patients with approximately 300 new cases being diagnosed each year. The mucus secreted by the membranes that line the airways and the gut is abnormally sticky with the result that the lungs are progressively damaged, digestion is impaired and the patient fails to thrive. The condition is due to a defect in a gene often called the 'cystic fibrosis gene', which directs the production of an essential protein. Since the identification and isolation of the cystic fibrosis gene in 1989, efforts have concentrated on developing techniques for inserting accurate copies of the gene into the patient's cells.

The aim of the research proposal was to develop a system to get the active gene, produced artificially in the laboratory, into the cells of the patient's nose and lungs where it would replace the function of the defective gene. The proposed method was to incorporate the manufactured gene into fatty droplets, known as liposomes. These would be inhaled by the patients in the hope that they would fuse with the membranes of the cells lining the respiratory tract and allow the genes to pass across into the cells. If successful, the replacement gene would then direct the production of the essential protein.

Severe combined immune deficiency syndrome

Severe combined immune deficiency (not to be confused with AIDS) is a rare inherited disorder in which the immune system is progressively damaged. The disorder arises as a result of a defective gene that in healthy individuals directs the production of an enzyme called adenosine deaminase. The disease was one of the first targets for gene therapy in the USA, two children undergoing gene therapy in 1990. It is an extremely rare disorder affecting only about five infants each year in the UK.

In the UK in 1993, the Committee on the Ethics of Gene Therapy approved a protocol in which a patient with the enzyme deficiency was to be treated by gene therapy. Bone marrow cells were removed, grown in the laboratory and then infected with a retrovirus carrying the normal human adenosine deaminase gene. The bone marrow cells receiving the normal gene from the virus were then returned to the child.

The research team reported that the gene was still found in the bone marrow six months after therapy, but unfortunately was not detected after one year. This is a promising start and it may be that further research will enable the technique to be used for the treatment of adenosine deaminase deficiency.

Research on cystic fibrosis and severe combined immune deficiency are two examples of the most straightforward application of gene therapy – the replacement of a defective gene by a good one. Although they are the most obvious applications of gene therapy, direct replacement studies of this kind accounted for less than 20 per cent of the first 100 proposals for gene therapy approved in the USA.

Imaginative applications of gene therapy

Most proposals were for projects aimed at obtaining a greater understanding of the processes involved in the development and treatment of cancer, using a variety of imaginative techniques. One example of a study considered in the UK by the Gene Therapy Advisory Committee is the injection into breast tumours of a plasmid with an attached gene coding for an enzyme that will convert an inactive drug into its active toxic form. In this way it is hoped that the drug will kill the cancer cells, without harming normal body cells.

Another study concerns a particular kind of lymphoma, where high dose chemotherapy may be beneficial, but cannot easily be used because of the damage it causes to bone marrow cells. The aim of the proposal was to remove bone marrow cells from the patient, introduce a gene coding for a protein that makes them resistant to the chemotherapy drugs, and then return them to the patient. As the modified bone marrow cells would now be resistant to its harmful effects, the hope is that it would then be possible to use higher dose chemotherapy.

These and other ingenious approaches to improving the treatment of cancer and other diseases may eventually yield worthwhile results, but their highly experimental nature means that they can only at present be used *in addition* to standard treatment. In such an exciting area of research, strict controls are required to ensure that some investigators do not allow their imagination to run away with them and embark on trials with a negligible chance of success.

By the end of 1995, in the UK, 55 patients had been recruited into nine studies (Gene Therapy Advisory Committee 1996, p.5). In the USA, 125 proposals for research on gene therapy had been approved up to October 1995, although only about half had started recruiting. Approximately 70 per cent of the studies related to cancer. At least 12 other studies were known by the Gene Therapy Advisory Committee (1996, p.7) to have been started, outside the UK and USA.

Germ-line gene therapy

The type of gene therapy that we have been considering, where a defective gene is replaced by a normal one in the lungs or blood cells, will only help the individual receiving the treatment. If the patient has children, the defective gene is still there to be passed onto them. In the future, gene modification of sperm or ova, or the cells that produce them, might prevent defective genes being transmitted to subsequent generations. Gene modification at an early stage of embryonic development might also be a way of correcting gene defects in both the germ-line and body cells. Such attempts are, however, fraught with danger and the Gene Therapy Advisory Committee has concluded that there is as yet insufficient knowledge to evaluate the risks to future generations.

The Clothier committee (Clothier 1992) recommends, therefore, that gene modification of the germ-line should not yet be attempted in humans.

18

Research on fetuses

The report of the Committee to Review the Guidance on the Research Use of Foetuses and Foetal Material, known as The Polkinghorne Report published in 1989, has become the standard source of guidance on the use of fetal tissue in the UK (Polkinghorne et al. 1989). On its publication, the government announced that they had accepted the Committee's main recommendations.

In such a sensitive area of research, however, it would be unrealistic to expect everyone to agree fully with all of its recommendations. Indeed, people who believe that abortion is unethical may well take the view that research on aborted fetuses is unethical, and it therefore follows that the production of guidelines on the use of such tissue is also unethical. The use of the term 'fetus' may also be regarded as dehumanising. Most women looking forward to the birth of a child will regard what they are carrying, not as a fetus, but as an unborn baby, while many couples go on to keep a copy of an ultrasound scan in their photograph album as the first photograph of their son or daughter.

Studies involving fetuses

The Polkinghorne report (Polkinghorne et al. 1989) emphasises that all research or therapy involving the fetus or fetal tissue must be described in a protocol and be examined by an ethics committee. Before approving the research, the committee must satisfy itself:

- ▶ of the validity of the research;
- ▶ that the objectives of the proposed use cannot be achieved in any other way;
- ▶ that the researchers or clinicians have the necessary facilities and skill.

Research on fetuses universally regarded as unethical

The Polkinghorne report (Polkinghorne et al. 1989) identifies certain kinds of research on the fetus which are always unethical and must never be permitted.

- ▶ It is unethical to administer any drugs or carry out any procedures during pregnancy with the intention of ascertaining whether or not they might harm a fetus which is later to be aborted (s.3.3).
- ▶ In the case of nervous tissue, only isolated cells or fragments of tissue may be used for transplantation (s.3.11).
  (There is a body of opinion that is totally opposed to the transfer of any kinds of nervous tissue from a fetus to an adult or to an animal.)
- ▶ In any study on human fetuses, the decision to terminate a pregnancy and the method and timing of the abortion must *not* be influenced by consideration of the possible uses that will be made of the tissue. This is also emphasised by the US regulations (45 CFR, 46.206a3).
  (The method used for bringing about the abortion will affect the usefulness of any tissue for research purposes. Suction evacuation of the uterus for instance disrupts the fetus making it difficult to isolate brain tissue, while prostaglandin-induced abortion damages pancreatic islet cells making them less suitable for transplantation experiments into the treatment of diabetes. Such considerations may create the temptation to select that abortion

technique which will result in fetal tissue satisfactory for a specific
research purpose.)

▶ The generation of pregnancy, or its termination, to produce
suitable tissue is unethical (s.4.1).
(The nightmare scenario was portrayed in an American hospital TV
drama where a fetus had been deliberately conceived in order to
provide nervous tissue to treat Parkinson's disease in its father.)

Separation of the source of tissue from the research

To reduce the risk of any stage of the abortion process being
influenced by the demands of the research, the Polkinghorne
report requires that medical staff who are involved in bringing
about the abortion and are responsible for the clinical care of the
mother should not themselves be involved with the subsequent use
of the fetal tissue (Polkinghorne et al. 1989, s.5.7). The US regulations also emphasise the importance of this (45 CFR, 46.206 a3).

The ideal method of separation is for a national tissue bank to
receive tissue and subsequently supply it to researchers. In the UK,
the Medical Research Council's fetal tissue bank at the
Hammersmith Hospital serves this purpose, and researchers who
can do their research on frozen tissue should obtain it from this
source. Where fresh tissue is required, a local mechanism will need
to be put into place that adequately separates the source of the
tissue from its use. This means designating an independent intermediary to receive and examine the fetal tissue before passing it on
to the appropriate researcher. The local research ethics committee
will need to satisfy itself on the adequacy of the system before it can
consider giving approval to a project involving fetal tissue.

Similarly, the determination of the death of the fetus should be
made or confirmed by a doctor responsible for the clinical care of
the mother and the fetus who is not involved with the research. In
the USA, the Code of Federal Regulations (45 CFR, 46.210) states that
'activities involving the dead fetus, macerated fetal material, or
cells, tissues or organs excised from a dead fetus shall be conducted

only in accordance with any applicable State or local laws regarding such activities'.

Potential uses to which tissue from a fetus may be put

The ethics of fetal research do not end with the question of whether or not aborted tissue should be used for research and how it should be obtained. The wide range of research uses to which tissue may be put raise ethical issues in their own right. The Polkinghorne report offers no guidance on this.

Homogenisation and chemical extraction

In many studies the tissue is homogenised and enzymes and other components extracted and investigated. This does not appear to raise additional ethical problems.

Culture of fetal tissue

More complex ethical problems arise when fetal tissue is to be cultured. Culturing means that the cells will be kept alive and allowed to multiply in flasks containing a solution of nutrients and growth factors. The result may be a cell line that will be in existence for many years after the fetus has been aborted. The culture of brain cells raises special ethical concerns.

Recent developments in cloning sheep suggest that it may theoretically be possible to use fetal cells for producing humans with the same genetic constitution as the original fetus (Wilmut et al. 1997). The potential use of fetal ova in assisted reproduction also raises major ethical concerns.

Transplanting tissue from a human fetus into animals

Serious ethical problems arise when it is proposed to graft living tissue from an otherwise dead fetus onto the body of a living animal. Many people would find such experimentation repugnant. Can there ever be a valid reason for doing it?

Let us consider the example of a research project where it is proposed to carry out fetal–animal transplants. A chemical has been identified that can give rise to cancer of the intestines. Investigators have fed this chemical to mice and found that there is an enzyme in the mouse intestine that can alter and detoxify the chemical, and that the activity of the enzyme is enhanced by the chemical itself and by vitamin supplements. To repeat the study in humans is obviously out of the question. So, in order to investigate whether the cancer-producing chemical and vitamins also enhance the activity of the equivalent enzyme in human intestine, they propose to take pieces of human intestine from an aborted fetus and graft it onto a mouse. The chemical can then be given to the mouse to see whether it increases the activity of the enzymes in the grafted human intestine as well as in mouse intestine.

The motives for doing the work may be high, but does the end (assuming the results are meaningful) justify the means? An ethics committee would be within its rights to say no if that was the feeling of its members. It would need to ask whether there were alternative methods of achieving the same end. Could pieces of adult intestine left over from an operation be used instead; or would the ultimate aim be better achieved by identifying the sources of the carcinogen and eliminating it from the environment, whilst encouraging a healthy vitamin rich diet.

Therapeutic research

Tissue from aborted fetuses has also been used in therapeutic research, the best known example being the use of fetal brain cells in an attempt to treat Parkinson's disease. Fetal thymus, pancreatic and liver cells have also been transferred to patients.

Informed consent for research on aborted fetuses

No one would deny the importance of obtaining the written consent of the mother before using her fetus for research. The Polkinghorne report states that: 'The consent of the mother must be obtained before any research or therapy involving the fetus or fetal tissue takes place. Sufficient explanation should be offered to make the act of consent valid' (Polkinghorne et al. 1989, s.6.3).

The report, however, also states that: 'The mother should not be informed of the specific use which may be made of fetal tissue, or whether it is to be used at all' (Polkinghorne et al 1989, s.4.2,4.6). This raises the question of how consent can be valid if the uses to which the tissue may be put are not clearly stated. Some women may be willing to allow enzymes to be extracted from dead tissue, but would be against the culture of live fetal cells or the transplantation of fetal tissue into animals. To do research of a nature which the mother may never have envisaged when giving her consent, and to which she may have been opposed, is surely unethical and contrary to Article I. 9 of the Declaration of Helsinki (World Medical Association 1996) which requires that: 'each potential subject must be adequately informed of the aims, methods, anticipated benefits, and potential hazards of the study.'

Obtaining specific consent could, however, undermine the central principle of the need for separation of the source of the fetus from the research. One compromise would be to give women a consent form listing various broad categories of research which they could consent to individually by means of a tick in the appropriate box, for example: (a) extraction of chemicals; (b) tissue culture; (c) prenatal diagnosis; (d) transplantation into animals; (e) transplantation into humans. If, therefore, the boxes permitting the use of the fetus for transplantation have not been ticked but the one allowing chemicals to be extracted has been, the fetal material could then be made available to the most relevant research group, but to no other.

Avoiding inducements

It is of the utmost importance that the decision to terminate a pregnancy should have been made *before* any reference is made to the possibility of the fetus being used in research (Polkinghorne et al. 1989, s.6.5). The decision to have an abortion must in no way be influenced by the thought that it might help in the quest for a treatment for a debilitating disease.

The separation of the source of the fetus from the researcher, as required by the Polkinghorne report, reduces the possibility of women being offered an inducement to allow their fetuses to be used in research. An inducement need not be financial – for example in some countries it could be the offer of an anaesthetic where abortions are normally performed without one. Inducements to mothers, whether financial or otherwise, to permit the use of their fetuses, or to doctors to obtain them, is unethical (Polkinghorne et al. 1989, s.4.4), as is profit derived from any dealing in fetal tissue (Polkinghorne et al. 1989, s.8.1, 8.3).

Should the father's consent be obtained?

The Polkinghorne committee considered that while it might be considered appropriate to consult the father, 'his consent should not be required, nor should he have the power to forbid research or therapy making use of fetal tissue' (Polkinghorne et al. 1989, s.6.7). This is a contentious statement, as it could be forcibly argued that ethically the father should have equal rights with the mother. He may have religious or moral beliefs that the mother does not have, and may have been opposed to the abortion in the first place. In research with babies or children, few researchers would wish to go ahead if the father disapproved, even if the consent of the mother (and of the child if mature enough) had already been obtained. An obvious exception would be if the conception was the result of rape.

Spontaneous abortions

Although the Polkinghorne report offers little advice on spontaneous abortions, it would seem wise only to approach women who are having elective abortions for social reasons. In view of the distress it could cause, it would not normally be considered ethical to approach a woman who had just suffered a spontaneous abortion of a much-wanted baby for permission to use it for research.

This should only be considered if the research is directly aimed at determining the cause of and preventing such abortions in other women, or possibly in a society where social abortions are not permitted. In the case of impending spontaneous abortions, consent to use the tissue, in the rare cases where this might be acceptable, should not be sought until after the fetus has died (Polkinghorne et al. 1989, s.6.7).

Similarly, a woman having an abortion because of a genetic defect found during prenatal screening, or for other medical reasons, is likely to be in an extremely distressed state and no effort should be made to make use of her fetus for research unless it is directly related to the condition concerned.

The involvement of mothers having live births in studies on aborted fetuses

Naturally enough, this eventuality was not perceived by the Polkinghorne report. As it may not be immediately apparent how this bizarre situation could arise, let us consider the example of a serious gastrointestinal problem of very premature babies. This problem appears to be due to the lack of a protective substance in the premature infant's gut, the production of which in full-term babies is stimulated by the mother's milk. In order to determine whether milk really does stimulate the production of this protective substance, it is proposed to treat slices of intestine taken from an aborted fetus with breast milk from a healthy mother.

The donation of a few millilitres of breast milk may in itself be regarded as a trivial request. But can it be assumed that a healthy mother would still be willing to donate her milk if she knew that the experiments involved aborted fetuses? Fully informed consent is, therefore, essential.

Obtain separate consent for HIV testing

Hepatitis and HIV testing of fetal material is routinely carried out if it is to be used for transplantation. As a positive result would have serious implications for the parents, their specific consent to testing must be obtained before being carried out. Similarly, if testing for hereditary disease is to be done on the fetus, both parents should first be consulted.

Withdrawal of consent – special problems

It is a well established principle that in obtaining consent for a procedure it should always be made clear to the patient that participation in the project is entirely voluntary and that either they may refuse to participate or they may withdraw at any time without giving a reason and without it affecting their future medical care. Most ethics committees require wording to this effect to be included in both the patient information sheet and consent form. In most types of research the implications of this are fairly straightforward. The patient starts off in a drug trial and then decides not to take the drug, or on seeing the actual questionnaire decides not to fill it in. The implications with fetal tissue research may be more far reaching.

If 'withdraw at any time' is to mean what it says, the mother could withdraw consent for the fetal tissue to be used, even after it had been taken, and the tissue could not then be used. If it had been, for example, transplanted into an animal the experiment would have to be terminated, or if a cell line had been established from the tissue this would then have to be destroyed, regardless of the research projects which currently depended on its use. The later the delay in withdrawing consent, the greater the potential problems. However, the option to 'withdraw at anytime' would not be feasible if the tissue had been used in the treatment of other people.

Other considerations

Conscientious objections amongst staff

To quote the Polkinghorne Report: 'No member of the medical or nursing staff should be under any duty to participate in research or therapy involving the fetus or fetal tissue if he or she has conscientious objections' (Polkinghorne et al. 1989, s.2.11). I trust that the authors of the Report would not object if this were extended to include scientific staff. Before approving a research proposal involving aborted fetuses, the medical research ethics committee will wish to obtain assurance that no member of staff will be pressurised into participating in the research if that individual does not wish to.

Preserving confidentiality

Maintaining confidentiality is vital in studies using aborted material. In a small town, there is every possibility that the young people working in the laboratory may have been to the same school as the woman undergoing the abortion and recognise the name on the sample. The record with the patient's personal details should be kept at source on the ward itself, with only a code number accompanying the fetal tissue to the laboratory. Consent forms should be kept securely locked away.

Embryo research

There is a body of opinion that regards all research on human embryos as unethical on the basis that, in the words of a statement issued in 1996 by the Centre of Bioethics at the Catholic University of the Sacred Heart in Rome (Instituto di Bioetica 1996):

> Embryos are human beings from the first moment they are
> formed, with a full personal individuality, and are able to develop
> completely, even if they are temporarily frozen.

The embryos that researchers wish to use are usually 'spare' embryos produced during in vitro fertilisation which, because the intended recipient does not need them anymore, are not destined to be transferred into her uterus, and are not required for donation to another woman.

Some investigators have asked to be allowed to perform experiments not only on spare embryos, but on embryos created specifically for experimentation, so that they can obtain a greater quantity of 'biological material' which is not altered by the process of freezing and thawing. It would seem a reasonable supposition that most people, even those not opposed to the use of 'spare' embryos, would question the ethics of the production of embryos specially for research. The creation of human embryos for research purposes is prohibited by Article 18.2 of the Convention for the Protection of Human Rights and Dignity of the Human Being with Regard to the Application of Biology and Medicine (Council of Europe 1997).

Licences for embryo research

In the UK, research which involves the creation, keeping or using of human embryos outside the body is governed by and must be licensed by the Human Fertilisation and Embryology Authority under the (1990) Human Fertilisation and Embryology Act (Morgan and Lee 1990). A centre must apply to the Authority for a separate licence for each research project.

Purposes allowed by the Human Fertilisation and Embryology Authority

Licences for research projects may be granted for the following purposes:

- ► To promote advances in the treatment of infertility.
- ► To increase knowledge about the causes of congenital diseases.
- ► To increase knowledge about the causes of miscarriages.
- ► To develop more effective techniques of contraception.
- ► To develop methods for detecting the presence of gene or chromosome abnormalities in embryos before implantation.

The Authority will grant a licence only if it is satisfied that the use of human embryos is essential for the purposes of the research. The scientific validity of all research projects involving the use of embryos must first be established by peer review undertaken by appropriate academic referees chosen by the Authority.

Activities NOT allowed
The following activities, as well as being unethical, are prohibited by UK law:

▶ Keeping or using an embryo after the appearance of the primitive streak or after 14 days, whichever is the earlier.
▶ Placing a human embryo in a non-human animal.
▶ Replacing a nucleus of a cell of an embryo with a nucleus taken from the cell of another person, another embryo, or a subsequent development of an embryo.
▶ Altering the genetic structure of any cell while it forms part of an embryo.

The researchers must refer each research project to a properly constituted ethics committee for approval before applying for a research licence. Membership of the ethics committee should be approved by the Authority to ensure that it contains a satisfactory mix of members who do not have a vested interest in this kind of research.

But is it ethical?

The groups and individuals opposed to research on human embryos will point out that the granting of a licence by the Human Fertilisation and Embryology Authority in UK, or equivalent bodies elsewhere, does not make such research ethical. They will argue that it is equally unethical to perform experiments on embryos up to 14 days as it is after 14 days. Fourteen days was taken as the limit by the Authority because after about the 14th day there is no longer the possibility that monozygotic twins can be produced from a single embryo. The embryo is then considered to be a single individual rather than potentially two individuals as before (Warnock 1984).

The simple truth of the matter is that no one can say exactly when a human life begins, so it can be argued that it is better to err on the side of ethical caution and assume that it begins at the moment of fertilisation.

Even with the approval of the Human Fertilisation and Embryology Authority and the local medical research ethics committee, research on spare embryos must *not* be done without the parents' informed consent. As this is an area where spiritual and religious convictions are paramount, it is of the utmost importance that the decision whether or not to consent to the use of their 'spare' embryos should be made free of any persuasive bias, such as a sense of gratitude to staff.

Even if all agree to participate in a particular case, this should not be allowed to create a precedent, as it still does not resolve the central question of whether it is ethical to conduct experiments on human embryos.

Cloning

The much publicised experiments of Wilmut and colleagues at the Roslin Research Institute near Edinburgh have demonstrated that the cloning of mammals is a possibility (Wilmut et al. 1997). There is no obvious reason why human tissue should behave very differently from that of sheep, so the cloning of an adult human could become feasible using the techniques perfected for sheep or other animals. While much of the speculation on the potential applications of the technology to humans has been in the realms of science fiction, there may be circumstances where cloning would be seriously considered. One situation is where the male partner is unable to produce functional sperm. A nucleus from one of his adult cells inserted into one of his wife's oocytes could theoretically give rise to a child with his genetic constitution (Kahn 1997; Winston 1997). Since, however, both sets of genes would then come from the man, the woman would be contributing little more genetically to their child than if she were a surrogate carrying an egg from another woman. The more traditional option of sperm donation when faced with an infertile male partner, though not without ethical problems of its own, would seem to be more in the woman's interest.

For it to be proved feasible, human cloning would need to undergo an experimental phase. It took scientists at the Roslin Institute 277 sheep eggs before they produced a live cloned lamb – a superovulated woman only produces five. You would therefore need a lot of superovulated women to do this and up to about 50 surrogate mothers. A large number of these would end in terminated pregnancies, and even among those that went full-term there would be a number of abnormalities. For all these reasons it would be unethical and extremely unwise to try human cloning (Bulfield 1998).

If it is universally regarded as unethical, now is the time to make the decision that human cloning will not be allowed under any circumstances. The Advisors to the President of the European Commission on the Ethical Implications of Biotechnology (1997) recommended that the European Commission should express its condemnation of human reproductive cloning, and the European Parliament has adopted a resolution forbidding such cloning (Anon, 1997b). In the USA, the National Bioethics Advisory Commission (1997) in its Report to President Clinton concluded that, 'at this time it is morally unacceptable for anyone in the public or private sector, whether in a research or clinical setting, to attempt to create a child using somatic cell nuclear transfer cloning', but legislation has yet to follow.

19

Animal to human transplantation

The Nuffield Council on Bioethics (NCB) set up a working party to address the issues raised by animal to human transplantation. Its report, *Animal to Human Transplants, the Ethics of Xenotransplantation,* published in 1996 provides a thorough account of the issues involved and is recommended to anyone with an interest in this area of research (NCB 1996). Some of the key issues relating to animal to human transplants raised by the Report are discussed below.

The practicalities

It will help to put the ethical issues into context if we first consider the practicalities of animal to human transplantation.

The key question is whether or not it can ever be made to work. One kind of animal to human transplant which is now routine is the use of pig heart valves to replace the patient's own defective valves. At the time of writing, however, attempts to replace whole human hearts, or other failing organs, such as the liver or kidneys with transplanted animal organs have met with little success.

The choice of species

Several major technical problems have to be overcome. Firstly, there is that of organ rejection. Even when an organ from another human being is transplanted, the recipient's immune system attacks the organ and immunosuppressive drugs have to be used to subdue the response. Not surprisingly, organ rejection becomes an even greater problem with animal to human grafting because of the greater difference between human and animal tissue. The more distantly related, in a biological sense, the human recipient is to the source animal, the stronger the immune reaction.

Primate organs

Attempts have been made in the USA to use organs from primates, such as baboons, for transplantation. Several ethical objections against the use of higher primates for transplantation have been raised including their closeness to human beings and capacity for self-awareness, and the possibility of increased pressure being placed on an already endangered primate population. A serious health risk associated with using primate organs for transplantation is that of introducing new diseases into the human population. The report of the UK government's Advisory Group on the Ethics of Xenotransplantation (1997) states that the use of primates is ethically unacceptable.

Pig organs

Many people would find the use of pigs more acceptable than that of primates, regarding a pig's capacity for self-awareness as being less (although some would disagree with this reasoning) and domestic pigs are in no danger of extinction. It is likely that a society that accepts the breeding of pigs for food and clothing would also accept their use for life-saving medical procedures. Pig organs are comparable in size to those of humans. Pigs reproduce quickly and produce large numbers of offspring.

The first question is whether a pig organ will be able to perform the functions that a healthy human organ does. The heart is a relatively simple mechanical pump, so an animal heart, in principle, should be able to perform the same function as a human heart. Other organs, notably the liver, have extremely complicated biochemical functions which differ between species. Proteins produced by a pig liver for instance may be functionally incompatible with those of a human recipient, and at the present time it is not known whether a non-human liver will support human life.

The second problem is the violent immune response to pig organs, which results in complete destruction of the transplanted organ, often in less than an hour. One promising approach for preventing organ rejection involves modifying the pig organs so that they do not cause such a strong immune response when transplanted into humans. This is done by altering the genetic make up of the pig by introducing human genetic material to produce so-called transgenic pigs. There is evidence from experiments with animal recipients that this approach can result in a reduction of the immune response when transgenic pig organs or tissues are transplanted into other species.

Thirdly, differences in life span must be considered. The natural life span of the pig is about 20 years. Would a transplanted pig organ age more rapidly than the human recipient? If so, this might lead to the need for successive transplants throughout the lifetime of the recipient. With so many technical problems, even if animal to human transplants are deemed to be ethical in other respects, the survival time of the early recipients is likely to be limited. A few animal to human transplants have been carried out since around 1964 but most patients have died within a few days.

Another potential advantage of using pigs is that, as they are less closely related to humans, the risk of introducing animal viruses and other disease agents into the human population is less, although with current concerns about the possibility of the agent that causes bovine spongiform encephalopathy (BSE) being transmitted from cattle to humans this argument may sound less convincing.

The possibility of viral transmission

There is a kind of influenza virus that is already known to affect both pigs and humans. In addition, pigs will be infected with microorganisms that do not normally infect humans. Transplantation of pig organs into humans may allow these microorganisms to infect the recipients, creating a previously unknown human disease.

As transplantation involves the direct introduction of animal organs or tissues into the human body, many of the natural barriers against infection are bypassed. Couple this with the fact that transplant recipients also require immunosuppressive drugs to prevent rejection of the transplant, which also have the effect of lowering the body's resistance to disease, and ideal conditions are created for the introduction of new viruses. That this is not pure speculation is emphasised by the observation that dogs, which are not normally susceptible to infection by a cat leukaemia virus can, following transplantation of infected cat tissue and administration of immuno-suppressive drugs, become infected with the virus and develop tumours (NCB 1996, s.6.7).

Some kinds of virus are very difficult to detect in the donor animals prior to transplanting their organs. One group, the retroviruses, remain hidden in the genetic material of the animal and can be passed from parent to off-spring. As there are likely to be many such viruses in pigs, which have yet to be identified (Allan 1997; Patience; Takeuchi and Weiss 1997), there is a risk that they will be transmitted to humans. There is also the risk that, without being able to harm the patient directly, an infectious organism present in the pig might cause disease in and destroy the transplanted organ. Even if virus-free when transplanted, the pig organ may remain susceptible to animal viruses. This is most likely to be a problem with lung transplants where infectious organisms of animals would easily gain access to the transplanted pig lung. Any person thinking about volunteering for animal to human transplants would have to be made aware of and to consider these risks, about which very little is known at present.

An even more serious possibility, which must be guarded against, is that should an animal virus infect a transplant patient, the resultant disease might then be passed onto the public at large.

In this way, animal to human transplants may pose a risk to public health as well to individual health.

Tissues which it may be unethical to transplant

Are there certain types of animal tissue which it is unethical to transplant into humans? A distinction may be drawn between material of a mechanical nature, such as heart muscle on the one hand, and brain cells on the other. Parkinson's disease sufferers have already received cells from the brain of a pig fetus in the hope that these will produce a substance in which sufferers from this disease are deficient (Deacon 1997). It must be said, however, that the issues raised by the use of human fetal tissue for this purpose are no less complex.

When will animal to human transplantation trials be justified?

By their nature, trials of new treatments involve unknown and unpredictable risks. It will not be known whether a pig kidney will function properly in a human body until the first transplants into humans are performed. Thus, even when the results from animal to animal experiments suggest that attempts at animal to human transplantation are justifiable these would still be a major and extremely risky operation. The UK government's Advisory Group on the Ethics of Xenotransplantation in its report published in 1997 did not regard it as ethically acceptable in the current state of knowledge to move to trials involving humans.

Facing a low chance of survival in the early stages

Experience with other major developments in medicine including human organ transplantation, the use of mechanical organs and, indeed, the few animal to human transplants already performed, suggest that early recipients will not have a good chance of survival. Any advances that are subsequently made are likely to be achieved at the expense of the first patients to be given the new treatment, some of whom may suffer a long, drawn out, painful death, instead of a relatively peaceful end.

On the other hand, there will be patients for whom the chance of making a contribution to medical research will provide a motive for accepting an animal organ. Respect for individual choice argues that people should be able to offer themselves as experimental subjects provided that adequate safeguards are in place to ensure that their consent is freely given and properly informed.

A central advisory committee

Among the recommendations of the Nuffield Council on Bioethics Working Party was the establishment of an advisory committee on animal to human transplantation, which would have the expertise to assess the success of species to species transplantation using animal models and to advise on when it is scientifically justified to begin clinical trials. Among its other functions would be the regulation of animal to human transplantation with respect to concerns about the possible transmission of disease-causing organisms.

Local research ethics committees would continue to review and approve proposals for research in this area. All such proposals would need to be approved by a local research ethics committee *in addition* to the approval of the proposed Advisory Committee on Animal to Human Transplantation. Experience of this kind of system is available from the field of gene therapy, trials of which require approval by the National Gene Therapy Advisory Committee as well as from local medical research ethics committees.

Following publication of the report of the UK government's Advisory Group on the Ethics of Xenotransplantation, *Animal Tissue into Humans* in 1997, the Health Secretary announced the setting up of an interim regulatory authority, pending primary legislation, to monitor all research into xenotransplantation.

The choice of first recipients

The working party stated that at first it would only be justifiable to offer animal organ transplantation if there was a reasonable chance of success and to patients for whom there was no alternative form of effective therapy. This would apply to some heart patients whose lives are at risk and for whom the shortage of human organs is acute. The lives of most kidney patients, however, can be maintained, albeit uncomfortably, on dialysis and they should not initially be offered such a high risk procedure (NCB 1996).

Children

The standard advice of the British Paediatric Association (1992), and other professional bodies that research should not be carried out on children if it could equally well be performed on adults applies as strongly here as elsewhere. With animal to human transplantation the main problem will be that of overcoming organ rejection which will affect all patients regardless of age. Until this problem is overcome in adults, the working party recommends that animal to human transplantation should not be attempted in children (NCB 1996, s.10.36).

Informed consent from transplant recipients

It is axiomatic that participants should give properly informed consent to any new treatment. They should be in a position to make a decision on the basis of proper information and without pressure, so that participation can be said to be truly voluntary. Patients are entitled to receive sufficient information in a way that they can understand about the proposed treatments, the possible alternatives and any substantial risks, so that they can make a balanced judgement. The problem is that the risks of animal to human transplantation will not be fully known until after a considerable number of operations have been carried out on humans. Patients must therefore be made aware of the extent to which they are experimental subjects involved in unpredictable clinical tech-niques that are largely in the developmental stages. The Nuffield Council on Bioethics Working Party recommended that the consent of patients to participation in animal to human transplan-tation trials should be obtained by trained professionals indepen-dent of the transplantation team. The information given to prospective recipients should include an estimation of the likely success, the risks and subsequent quality of life (NCB 1996, s.10.34).

Adults who cannot consent on their own behalf

The working party recommends that early transplantation trials should be restricted to adults capable of consenting to partic-ipation on their own behalf. Adults with learning disability should not be involved until the technology has been worked out (NCB 1996, s.10.38).

Follow-up of animal transplant recipients

There will be a need for continuous monitoring and surveil-lance of early recipients of animal transplant organs. Regular phys-ical examinations with storage of serum samples and/or tissue samples should continue throughout the lifetime of the recipient. Serum samples taken from health care workers caring for the recip-ient should also be archived. The recipient should be required to report any serious unexplained illness, as should family members and others who come into close contact with them. In addition, recipients should be urged to take routine precautions to minimise the transmission of infectious disease, such as not donating blood, and they should be counselled on methods of minimising trans-mission by sexual contact. The procedures to be followed should a disease be found to be transmitted from the donor animals to human recipients, need to be established.

In view of the importance of monitoring recipients for any evidence that diseases are being transmitted from animals to man, patients consenting to transplantation must be informed that post-operative monitoring is an essential part of the procedure and that their consent to the operation includes consent to this monitoring (NCB 1996, s.10.28). The customary right of patients to withdraw their consent at any time would need to be waived in this instance, withdrawal only being possible prior to the operation.

The working party recommended that a protocol to conduct a trial should be accepted only if it contains a commitment to provide a full description and assessment of the patients' pre-operative and post-operative quality of life (NCB 1996, s.10.35). Since animal to human transplantation will be an experimental procedure on every occasion on which it is undertaken in the near to medium term it is essential that those carrying out the procedure report fully on all important consequences.

Longer term implications for patients

Will refusal of animal organs compromise the right to other forms of treatment?

Should the technology prove feasible and animal to human transplantation enter into widespread use, patients must be entitled to decline such a transplant for any religious, cultural or ethical reason or indeed because they do not believe that the benefits outweigh the risks.

What are the implications for people who refuse animal to human transplants? If developed into a successful procedure it might offer a cheaper form of treatment, for example, than dialysis for patients with kidney failure, resulting in pressure on individuals to accept these grafts. How would refusal of an animal organ affect an individual's consideration for human organ transplantation? Could their priority for receiving a human organ be reduced on the grounds that they have been offered and refused an appropriate alternative form of treatment? This would undermine the concept of freely given consent. The working party recommends that at any stage in the development of animal to human transplantation, patients who, for whatever reasons, refuse animal transplants should remain entitled to consideration for human organs on the same basis as before their refusal (NCB 1996, s.10.40).

The question also arises as to what should happen to the patient who in the absence of a suitable human organ, has accepted an animal organ but for whom a human transplant at some later date might offer a better prognosis. Will the fact that they have already received the animal transplant relegate them to the bottom of the waiting list for human transplants? In practice, animal organ transplantation might be used as a bridging procedure to keep a patient alive until a human organ became available. The working party recommends that animal transplant recipients should remain entitled to consideration for human organ transplantation on the same basis of clinical need as before receiving the animal organ (NCB 1996, s.10.41). It recognises that the demand for human organs, instead of declining as a result of animal organs being used, may even increase in the early years of animal transplantation, since animal organ recipients may remain on the waiting list for human organs whereas, without an animal organ, they might not have survived. Ironically, there is a danger that inappropriate publicity concerning animal to human transplants may reduce the supply of human organs (NCB 1996, s.10.46).

The emotional impact

The emotional impact of animal organ transplants on recipients should also be studied. Some patients receiving human organs find it disturbing that they have inside them an organ from someone who has died. The working party recommends that counselling of animal organ recipients should include discussion of the possible personal impact of transplantation, and recommends that research should be initiated to study this (NCB 1996, s.10.45).

Conclusion

Animal to human transplantation clearly raises many ethical issues to tax the minds of the investigators, medical research ethics committees and society as a whole. In the light of so many problems, the first question to be resolved is whether it should be attempted at all.

20

Post-approval monitoring of
research by ethics committees

There is in general, widespread acceptance within society for monitoring of medical research. It is, therefore, remarkable that medical research ethics committees in countries like the UK have no formal mechanism in place to ensure that investigators are adhering to and meeting the conditions set by committees. Trials sponsored by pharmaceutical companies are an exception to this. Stringent monitoring of drug trials by appropriately trained monitors is a requirement of good clinical practice, the aim being to verify that: the rights and well-being of subjects are protected; the reported data are accurate, complete and verifiable from source documents; and that the conduct of the trial is in compliance with the currently approved protocol/amendments, with good clinical practice, and with the applicable regulatory requirements (International Conference on Harmonisation 1996, s.5.18). This process is now being audited by government regulatory bodies. Most studies not sponsored by pharmaceutical companies, however, still remain unmonitored following ethical approval.

There is a requirement in the USA for institutional review boards (IRBs) to conduct continuing review of all approved studies at intervals of not more than one year (45 CFR 46.109e; 21 CFR 56.109e). When the IRB conducts continuing review, it should review as a minimum, 'the protocol and any amendments, as well as a status report on the progress of the research, including: (a) the number of subjects accrued; (b) a description of any adverse events, or unanticipated problems involving risks to subjects or others, withdrawal of subject from the research or complaints about the research; (c) a summary of any recent literature, findings, or other relevant information, especially information about risks associated with the research; and (d) a copy of the informed consent document' (Office for Protection from Research Risks 1995). The regulations do not provide specific instructions to IRBs on how to perform continuing review, nor demand that this is conducted on site. It is however, emphasised that the official requirement should be seen as a minimum and IRBs are given the authority to observe or have a third party observe the consent process and the research (45 CFR, 46.109e).

In drug trials, continuing review by IRBs is complemented by the audits conducted by the Food and Drug Administration in an effort to detect professional misconduct. (Weiss et al. 1993).

Following implementation of the International Conference on Harmonisation, *Guideline for Good Clinical Practice* in January 1997, in the UK the Department of Health's Medicines Control Agency has set up a Good Clinical Practice Compliance Unit to monitor studies sponsored by pharmaceutical companies. Monitors will visit the companies and investigator sites. Currently the Unit has no authority to monitor the workings of ethics committees. In the USA, however, the Food and Drug Administration already conducts reviews to determine whether an IRB is operating in accordance with its own written procedures and with the FDA regulations (FDA Compliance Guidance Manual for IRB Inspections).The European Medicines Evaluation Agency is also embarking on a similar system of monitoring clinical trials.

The view of the medical profession in the UK in regard to continuing review of studies approved by local research ethics committees has been ambivalent. The Royal College of Physicians accept that local research ethics committees should not lose contact with investigations that they have approved and that some follow-up is desirable, but considers that, 'it is impracticable, even if it were desirable, for an ethics committee to monitor in detail the conduct of ongoing investigations (Royal College of Physicians 1996, s.2.12–2.13)'. The College recommends, however, that some sort of follow up is desirable and suggests an annual questionnaire to applicants to establish whether the project has been completed, abandoned or is still in progress and to obtain information on adverse events. It also suggests that in addition, a more detailed follow up of selected projects may be preferred. The difficulty of reviewing every project in detail after approval is also emphasised by the Royal College of Psychiatrists (1990).

Guidance from the Department of Health simply recommends that researchers should be required to inform local research ethics committees in advance of significant proposed deviations from the original protocol, and of any events which raise concern about the safety of the research (Department of Health 1991, s.2.14). The question that local research ethics committees have to address is: what practical arrangements should a committee make in order to satisfy itself that medical research studies are being conducted in accordance with the proposal forms, protocol, participant information sheets and consent forms that have been approved.

Monitoring of research by the Tayside Committee on Medical Research Ethics

As a literature search and contact with other ethics committees failed to reveal any instances of detailed on-site monitoring being currently practised by a UK committee, the Tayside Committee on Medical Research Ethics in Scotland, with a view to seeking an answer to this question, embarked on a pilot study to investigate the feasibility and effectiveness of on-site review of projects that they had previously approved (Smith, Moore and Tunstall-Pedoe 1997).

The methodology which has now been approved for routine monitoring in Tayside, is described below, and some observations made that may be of interest to other committees considering the possibility of embarking on the post approval review of projects.

The methodology

The ethics committee selects for review a stratified random sample of 10 per cent of the research studies approved approximately one year previously. A third of the sample is made up of studies sponsored by pharmaceutical companies with the remaining studies selected from university or health service initiated projects.

The assessors contact the researchers, explain the objective of the exercise and arrange a meeting. This involves two members of the ethics committee – one lay and one medically qualified. The meeting is confirmed by letter and a copy of a Questionnaire for Researchers sent prior to the meeting for researchers to complete. A copy of this questionnaire can be found in Appendix 7.

At each review meeting, the assessors:

- discuss the responses to the questionnaire for researchers;
- complete an assessors questionnaire for recording further details of the visit;
- inspect consent forms;
- inspect case records.

The following information is recorded on the questionnaires.

- Title of proposal.
- Date, time and place of review meeting.
- Names and titles of researchers present.
- Identification of any difficulties experienced in complying with the protocol.
- A summary of adverse events.
- The method of providing participants with information about the project and of obtaining consent.
- Any refusal by a patient or volunteer to take part in the study.
- Any withdrawal from the study.
- Whether or not a final report was or would be available for the ethics committee.

► Any comments made in explanation of responses to the above questions and any additional comments on any aspect of the monitoring visit.
► The number of consent forms available and the correctness of their completion.
► The number of case record forms examined and whether or not satisfactorily completed.

Data from the questionnaires is recorded on a database to facilitate analysis of the results. The assessors subsequently send a letter to researchers summarising the main points raised at the meeting and advising them of any modifications needed to meet the requirements of the committee. In the case of a serious breach of the rules, they will send copies of the letter to the researchers' head of department and head of their employing institutions.

Was the study begun on schedule?

The initial contact required to arrange a monitoring meeting usually reveals that a significant proportion of the proposals approved by the committee fail to get off the ground – some are abandoned due to lack of funding, others are still awaiting funding. Researchers often omit to inform the ethics committee if a study is abandoned or that there is a significant delay in starting. In view of this, we would recommend that a routine letter is sent annually to researchers asking them to advise the ethics committee of the status of their projects.

Concern for research participants

Assessors will wish to confirm that researchers are putting the well-being of patients or healthy volunteers before the requirements of the research protocols, as evidenced by them being unwilling to approach patients regarding participation if they think they are too ill to take them off medication on which they are stabilised or to use invasive procedures in their research when non-invasive methods are available. They should also be willing to withdraw patients from trials if it is in the patients' interests to do so.

Difficulties in recruitment

The monitoring meeting allows difficulties in recruitment to be identified. A common reason for recruitment difficulties in drug trials is that doctors do not wish to recruit patients who are stabilised on current treatment when there is no indication for a change with the result that patient numbers are restricted. Sponsors may terminate studies owing to insufficient patients having been recruited by the doctor for this reason within the required time. Competition from other research groups for certain groups of patients who are in high demand, such as those with asthma, may also pose a problem.

Maintaining the right to withdraw

It is important that research participants are fully aware of their right to withdraw from a study at any time and for whatever reason. Assessors need to establish how many patients have exercised this right and to discuss the reasons for their withdrawal. Did they decide unilaterally or in discussion with the researchers? Were any of the withdrawals due to unacceptable discomforts or side-effects of the treatment or to patients being dissatisfied with the way they had been treated by the staff?

It is equally important that researchers should be willing to withdraw patients if it does not seem in their best interests to continue. It will be reassuring to assessors to see that researchers withdraw patients for reasons such as lack of expected improvement in their condition, or the fact that they are experiencing too much pain from their condition to justify exposing them to further inconvenience. Rarer reasons for withdrawal may turn up, such as the early symptoms of Alzheimer's disease aggravated by a change of environment necessary for the study.

Compliance with the protocol

Amendments to the protocol

Investigators must comply with the approved protocol and notify all amendments to the committee for approval before implementing them. Monitoring provides the opportunity to check whether any changes have been made to the protocol and to ensure that this requirement has been adhered to. Failure to notify amendments such as changes to the dose of the study drug, or inclusion criteria, puts researchers in the unacceptable position of carrying out research which has not been ethically approved.

As one of the key roles of an ethics committee is to assess the suitability of the researchers to conduct the proposed research, assessors will need to check that the researchers have notified the committee prior to new researchers becoming involved in the project.

Reporting of adverse events

All serious adverse events must be reported to the ethics committee. The review meeting provides the opportunity to check that this is being done and to discuss with researchers the kind of adverse event that should be reported. Although those of a non-serious, but unpleasant, nature such as dizziness, drowsiness, diarrhoea, vomiting or heartburn need not be reported, anything more serious, whether believed to be related to the treatment or not, should be. The reporting of serious adverse events is considered in more detail in the section on clinical trials.

Availability of a study report

Research is of limited value if the results are not widely disseminated so that others can make use of the findings (Savulescu,

Chalmers and Blunt, 1996). The assessors will therefore be interested to see whether researchers are committed to publish the results of their research in national and international journals. The ability to get papers published is also an indication of the quality of the research, with the important proviso that it is often difficult to persuade professional journals to publish negative results despite their potential value.

Has fully informed consent been obtained?

A key purpose of monitoring is to ensure that researchers are obtaining informed consent from patients in all studies in which this is possible. In most studies, all of the participants will be potentially capable of giving consent. Any who are not, for example a patient with Alzheimer's disease who is encountered by chance at a diabetic clinic whilst recruiting for a study into diabetes, should not be included. In studies specifically aimed at improving the care of patients with Alzheimer's disease or other susceptible groups where their condition prevents patients from giving informed consent, the consent of relatives or trusted carers should have been obtained instead.

Assessors will also need to confirm that researchers are giving their patients the approved amount of time to decide whether to join the study as stated on the proposal form.

Availability and completeness of consent forms

As this stage of monitoring involves one or more ethics committee members in gaining access to confidential information about the patients – even if only their name – it is important that patients should have given permission for this. The possibility of the project being monitored by members of the ethics committee should therefore have been stated in the patient information sheet as part of the process of obtaining informed consent.

In preparation for the meeting, researchers should aim to have all of the consent forms available for scrutiny. Despite this, assessors may well find that consent forms are missing for any one of a variety of reasons. For example, they may be filed in hospital case notes which are in use elsewhere, verbal consent may have been obtained instead, a co-researcher may have taken them away to write up the study, they may have all been returned to the sponsor or just mislaid. Although not ethically so questionable, the legal consequences of the inability to produce a valid consent form could be as great as not having obtained one in the first place. When the researcher has not been involved in the consent procedure, as would be the case in, for example, a study involving aborted fetal tissue, the person who obtained consent should be present at the review meeting and bring the consent forms with them.

The Tayside Ethics Committee have observed instances where although the principle researcher always takes care to obtain informed consent, a collaborating researcher, who has not been adequately informed of its importance, may not have done so, particularly in non-invasive procedures where the researcher may not have seen the need. Assessors may need to remind researchers that while some studies may not involve invasive procedures or any risk to the subjects, it is still normally essential to obtain informed consent. They may still involve highly confidential information or the possibility of the diagnosis of previously unsuspected illness. Informed consent must always be obtained from participants even if, as in one study monitored, the subject is the researcher's supervisor!

Monitoring provides the opportunity to ensure that the consent given by patients is valid. In the case of the recommended consent form with the 'Yes:No' format of which there is an example in Appendix 5, the assessors will need to check that each question has been answered satisfactorily. Assessors often find that patients have for example, not answered all of the questions or have indicated that they have not seen the information sheet or not had the opportunity to ask questions, and yet the researchers have accepted their signature at the bottom of the form giving their consent. Consent forms may also be discovered that have not been countersigned by the doctor. The discovery of such errors provides assessors with the opportunity to emphasise to researchers the importance of carefully checking consent forms to ensure that participants have completed them correctly and are satisfied with the information provided before they countersign them and start the study.

Availability of case records

Examination of case records provides a means of assessing the thoroughness with which data relevant to the scientific validity of the study and the patients' welfare are being recorded. Research case records will not, however, be available for inspection if they are filed with the patient's hospital case notes which are in use elsewhere in the hospital. Some hospital case notes are extremely bulky and considerable difficulty may be experienced by the researchers and reviewers in finding the consent forms and other records relevant to the study being reviewed.

If assessors find that there is a need for access to research case records to be improved, they should provide advice. Records relevant to a research project including the signed consent forms should be kept in a separate folder in the possession of the researcher, while a contact number and other essential details relating to the patient's involvement in the project is included, along with a copy of the information sheet and consent form, in the hospital case notes.

A common problem with case records of drug company studies is the lack of legibility of the copies retained by the researcher. This may be especially noticeable in studies involving patients with conditions such as rheumatoid arthritis, where their difficulty in applying sufficient pressure to give a legible copy may not have been taken into account by the pharmaceutical company in the design of their forms. Research case records should be scrutinised, as far as the expertise of the assessors allows, to determine if there are any errors in completion which might affect the validity of the studies.

Educational value of monitoring

Researchers have recently strongly criticised local medical research ethics committees on various grounds, which were summarised in a recent editorial (Alberti 1995) to which an experienced committee member replied with points in their favour (Tunstall-Pedoe 1995).

Despite the criticisms, and the uncertainty expressed by the professional bodies about the need for review after ethical approval has been given, the researchers we approached were, without exception, very supportive of the work of the committee and of the idea of post-approval ethical review. We trust that other committees which embark on post approval review will share our experience.

The educational value both for researchers and committee members of review meetings is considerable. Ethical review can inform the reviewers, and through them the whole committee, of the realities of a wide range of research procedures and identify key concerns that need to be addressed. This helps the committee in the scrutiny of new proposals that come before it, and contributes to the advice given to researchers with the proposal form and in the annual reports.

Awareness of the possibility of review after ethical approval provides an added incentive not to cut corners and to maintain standards, thereby helping to protect research participants from potential harm and investigators from criticism. It would also provide a further disincentive to potential research fraud, cases of which come to light from time to time (Smith 1996; Wells 1996; Dyer 1997; Wells and Blunt 1997).

Constructive feedback to the individual researchers is considered an essential part of the exercise and is likely to be appreciated by them. It should include a constructive letter detailing the main issues raised at the meeting and any adjustments required to conform to the requirements of the committee. The compulsory ethics committees' annual reports (Department of Health 1991 s.2.16; Nicholson 1997a) should be fully exploited as a means of communicating to the local research community points of general relevance raised during the review process, appropriately anonymised to protect the identity of the researchers and to offer guidance on those issues about which researchers express uncertainty.

A number of researchers have raised the question of seeking the views of patients and volunteers during and following their participation in research projects, reinforcing the Committee's belief in the importance of this aspect of monitoring.

The patient questionnaire

It may be preferable for questionnaires to be issued on behalf of the committee by the researcher. This will avoid patients getting the impression that the ethics committee is checking up on their doctor which may cause them to become protective and paint too rosy a picture. An opening line such as, 'The aim of the questionnaire is to help us to improve our service towards patients involved in research', establishes that the questionnaire is being put out with the researcher's approval. In order for patients to feel free to express their honest feelings the questionnaire must, however, assure them that their responses will only be seen by members of the ethics committee, and not be communicated to the doctor in a manner that could identify who made them.

A specimen patient questionnaire is given in Appendix 6.

An anonymised analysis of the responses needs to be fed back to the researchers concerned, with due regard for the anonymity of the patients, to enable them to identify any weaknesses in their relationship with participants, and to work out how best to improve them. In the event of the patients' responses giving rise to serious concerns by the ethics committee about the conduct of the research, the researcher should be requested to report back to the committee with details of how the problems raised are going to be tackled. Identification of specific problems, as well as being of benefit to the researcher, will enable the ethics committee to identify areas where problems can sometimes arise so that advice can be offered to all researchers.

The cost of ethical review

The costs of ethical review are significant. A review visit involves about six person hours of work for the assessors. In addition, an hour of the researchers' time for the visit and additional preparation time must be taken into account. The review of proposals after approval should be brought into the discussion regarding the charging of commercial companies.

Conclusion

Public confidence in medical research and the willingness to co-operate will continue only if the research is seen to be conducted to the highest ethical standards demanded by government and international regulations and professional bodies (e.g. 45 CFR 46; 21 CFR 50 and 56; CIOMS/WHO 1993; ICH 1996; RCP 1996). The existence of an effective system for the review of research demonstrates that efforts are being made to maintain these high standards. While ethics committees in the UK do not have the authority to take direct action against researchers guilty of serious misconduct, such as repeated failure to obtain informed consent for no good reason, they may report researchers to their employing authority and professional bodies who will then consider what further action is appropriate. Under the International Committee on Harmonisation (1996, s.5.20.2) guidelines, pharmaceutical company monitors/auditors must inform both the local ethics committee and the regulatory authorities if a trial is stopped at a centre in their area due to persistent non-compliance with good clinical practice by the investigator.

While the primary aim of post approval review is to protect patients, it is also of positive value to researchers, many of whom are working in a vacuum and welcome a forum for discussion to ensure that their procedures are seen as satisfactory. Public expectations and accountability are constantly increasing and in these days of investigative journalism and litigation for negligence, researchers also need to ensure that they are not inadvertently leaving themselves open to criticism.

The importance of the monitoring of research projects was recently emphasised in a Sheriff's report of a fatal accident inquiry in Scotland following the death of a research participant. The report stated, 'it is clearly not satisfactory that there was no mechanism in place for a much closer monitoring of research projects such as that by the ethics committee which would have prevented this [*the failure to obtain proper consent*] happening and that is a matter which should be addressed as a matter of urgency.' (Sheriff's Report, 1997).

Our experience of monitoring leads us to recommend that all local medical research ethics committees should randomly select a minimum of ten per cent of approved projects, and any additional projects which arouse specific concerns, for subsequent on-site review by members of the committee. In addition, specific studies that cause particular concern should be monitored as determined by the committee. We recommend that all remaining projects should be reviewed by questionnaire and that a sample of patients should also be asked to complete a questionnaire about their participation, to assess their satisfaction with how they were treated.

► Appendix 1
World Medical Association – Declaration of Helsinki

Recommendations guiding physicians in biomedical research involving human subjects.

Adopted by the 18th World Medical Assembly, Helsinki, Finland, June 1964; amended by the 29th World Medical Assembly, Tokyo, October 1975; the 35th World Medical Assembly, Venice, Italy, October 1983; the 41st World Medical Assembly, Hong Kong, September 1989; and the 48th General Assembly, Somerset West, Republic of South Africa, October 1996.

Introduction

It is the mission of the physician to safeguard the health of the people. His or her knowledge and conscience are dedicated to the fulfilment of this mission.

The Declaration of Geneva of the World Medical Association binds the physician with the words, 'The health of my patient will be my first consideration,' and the International Code of Medical Ethics[1] declares that, 'A physician shall act only in the patient's interest when providing medical care which might have the effect of weakening the physical and mental condition of the patient.'

The purpose of biomedical research involving human subjects

---

1 Because the language of the Hippocratic Oath is archaic, a modernised version was introduced in 1947 by the World Medical Association known as the Declaration of Geneva. It was amended in Sydney in 1968 and in Venice in 1983 and now forms the basis of the International Code of Medical Ethics. (World Medical Association 1993).

must be to improve diagnostic, therapeutic and prophylactic procedures and the understanding of the aetiology and pathogenesis of disease.

In current medical practice most diagnostic, therapeutic or prophylactic procedures involve hazards. This applies especially to biomedical research.

Medical progress is based on research which ultimately must rest in part on experimentation involving human subjects.

In the field of biomedical research, a fundamental distinction must be recognised between medical research in which the aim is essentially diagnostic or therapeutic for a patient, and medical research, the essential object of which is purely scientific and without implying direct diagnostic or therapeutic value to the person subjected to the research.

Special caution must be exercised in the conduct of research which may affect the environment, and the welfare of animals used for research must be respected.

Because it is essential that the results of laboratory experiments be applied to human beings to further scientific knowledge and to help suffering humanity, the World Medical Association has prepared the following recommendations as a guide to every physician in biomedical research involving human subjects. They should be kept under review in the future. It must be stressed that the standards as drafted are only a guide to physicians all over the world. Physicians are not relieved from criminal, civil and ethical responsibilities under the laws of their own countries.

Basic principles

(1) Biomedical research involving human subjects must conform to generally accepted scientific principles and should be based on adequately performed laboratory and animal experimentation and on a thorough knowledge of the scientific literature.

(2) The design and performance of each experimental procedure involving human subjects should be clearly formulated in an

experimental protocol which should be transmitted for consideration, comment and guidance to a specially appointed committee independent of the investigator and the sponsor provided that this independent committee is in conformity with the laws and regulations of the country in which the research experiment is performed.

(3) Biomedical research involving human subjects should be conducted only by scientifically qualified persons and under the supervision of a clinically competent medical person. The responsibility for the human subject must always rest with a medically qualified person and never rest on the subject of the research, even though the subject has given his or her consent.

(4) Biomedical research involving human subjects cannot legitimately be carried out unless the importance of the objective is in proportion to the inherent risk to the subject.

(5) Every biomedical research project involving human subjects should be preceded by careful assessment of predictable risks in comparison with foreseeable benefits to the subject or to others. Concern for the interests of the subject must always prevail over the interests of science and society.

(6) The right of the research subject to safeguard his or her integrity must always be respected. Every precaution should be taken to respect the privacy of the subject and to minimise the impact of the study on the subject's physical and mental integrity and on the personality of the subject.

(7) Physicians should abstain from engaging in research projects involving human subjects unless they are satisfied that the hazards involved are believed to be predictable. Physicians should cease any investigation if the hazards are found to outweigh the potential benefits.

(8) In publication of the results of his or her research, the physician is obliged to preserve the accuracy of the results. Reports of experimentation not in accordance with the principles laid down in this Declaration should not be accepted for publication.

(9) In any research on human beings, each potential subject must be

adequately informed of the aims, methods, anticipated benefits and potential hazards of the study and the discomfort it may entail. He or she should be informed that he or she is at liberty to abstain from participation in the study and that he or she is free to withdraw his or her consent to participation at any time. The physician should then obtain the subject's freely-given informed consent, preferably in writing.

(10) When obtaining informed consent for the research project the physician should be particularly cautious if the subject is in a dependent relationship to him or her or may consent under duress.

In that case the informed consent should be obtained by a physician who is not engaged in the investigation and who is completely independent of this official relationship.

(11) In the case of legal incompetence, informed consent should be obtained from the legal guardian in accordance with national legislation. Where physical or mental incapacity makes it impossible to obtain informed consent, or when the subject is a minor, permission from the responsible relative replaces that of the subject in accordance with national legislation.

Whenever the minor child is in fact able to give consent, the minor's consent must be obtained in addition to the consent of the minor's legal guardian.

(12) The research protocol should always contain a statement of the ethical considerations involved and should indicate that the principles enunciated in the present Declaration are complied with.

Medical research combined with professional care (Clinical research)

(1) In the treatment of the sick person, the physician must be free to use a new diagnostic and therapeutic measure, if in his or her judgement it offers hope of saving life, re-establishing health or alleviating suffering.

(2) The potential benefits, hazards and discomfort of a new method should be weighed against the advantages of the best current diagnostic and therapeutic methods.

(3) In any medical study, every patient – including those of a control group, if any – should be assured of the best proven diagnostic and therapeutic method. This does not exclude the use of an inert placebo in studies where no proven diagnostic or therapeutic method exists.

(4) The refusal of the patient to participate in a study must never interfere with the physician–patient relationship.

(5) If the physician considers it essential not to obtain informed consent, the specific reasons for this proposal should be stated in the experimental protocol for transmission to the independent committee (1, 2).

(6) The physician can combine medical research with professional care, the objective being the acquisition of new medical knowledge, only to the extent that medical research is justified by its potential diagnostic or therapeutic value for the patient.

Non-therapeutic biomedical research involving human subjects (Non-clinical biomedical research)

(1) In the purely scientific application of medical research carried out on a human, it is the duty of the physician to remain the protector of the life and health of that person on whom biomedical research is being carried out.

(2) The subjects should be volunteers – either healthy persons or patients for whom the experimental design is not related to the patient's illness.

(3) The investigator or the investigating team should discontinue the research if in the investigator's or their judgement it may, if continued, be harmful to the individual.

(4) In research on humans, the interest of science and society should never take precedence over considerations related to the well-being of the subject.

Appendix 2
A specimen local medical research ethics committee constitution

(Name) Committee on Medical Research Ethics Constitution

Title

There shall be constituted a committee on medical research ethics of (NAME) health authority entitled the (NAME) Committee on Medical Research Ethics.

Functions

- The Committee will independently assess all applications to undertake research involving patients, volunteers, the recently dead, fetal material, waste tissue, and access to medical records; whether from hospital practice, the university, general practice, private practice or industry or other source, within its geographical area of authority.
- The Committee will encourage high ethical standards in all research referred to it for consideration.
- The first responsibility of the Committee will be to protect the mental and physical well-being and moral rights of the patients or volunteers involved, as detailed in the Declaration of Helsinki and subsequent amendments.
- The Committee will also have the responsibility of protecting the interests of researchers and of the health authority, hospitals, research institutions and university where any matter of an ethical

nature might affect these interests, provided that the interests of patients and volunteers take priority.

Membership

► The local medical research ethics committee shall comprise 12 members, each of whom shall be appointed by or on behalf of the local health authority after having consulted with relevant health service bodies, local professional advisory committees and patient organisations as appropriate. The health authority shall ensure, so far as possible, that the membership includes:

    (i) general representation of the major medical/clinical specialisation's practised within the authority;

    (ii) hospital medical staff, nursing staff, general practitioners, a pharmacist, a statistician and at least three lay persons.

The health professionals shall include those with experience in research and investigation as well as those involved in active clinical care. At least one of the lay members shall have no connection, past or present, with any health service body or medical research establishment either as an employee or an adviser (except as a lay member of an ethics committee). Membership of the local medical research ethics committee shall include representatives of both sexes, and a range of age groups. Members are appointed as 'individuals of sound judgement' and must not be seen as representing any professional or other group.

► Members shall serve for a period of three years, renewable for one further term.

► A member may resign from the Committee at any time upon giving notice in writing to the health authority. Membership will lapse if a member fails without excuse/notifying the chairperson to attend three consecutive meetings of the Committee. Steps shall be taken by or on behalf of the authority to fill, without undue delay, any vacancy that may arise.

► The health authority shall appoint a chairperson and a vice-chairperson of the committee after consultation with the committee members. The appointees shall normally be experienced ethics committee members. Either the chairperson or the vice-chairperson shall be lay members of the committee. In the absence of the chairperson, the vice-chairperson will perform the role and duties of chairperson to include taking chairperson's action and officiating at committee meetings.

► The committee may co-opt additional members as appropriate after consultation with the health authority.

► The health authority shall provide adequate administrative and secretarial support to the Committee.

Quorum

The minimum number constituting a quorum will be six, including at least one lay and two medically qualified members.

Members unable to attend a meeting are encouraged to submit detailed written comments on proposals, which will be considered at the meeting, but the normal requirement for six members present will still apply.

Criteria to be met in submitting applications to the committee

Submission in a standard format

Applications for ethical approval must be submitted to the secretary of the committee on the standard form approved by the committee, including the written information, questionnaires, etc., which it is intended to supply to patients. Studies previously submitted to a multicentre research ethics committee will, however, be accepted on the multicentre committee's standard proposal form. The number of copies required by the committee must be submitted in all cases.

Informed consent

The research subjects must be adequately informed of the aims, methods, anticipated benefit and potential hazards of the study, including any discomfort it might entail and any costs they may have to bear (e.g., extra visits to hospital). They must be aware of their right to decline to participate and to leave the study at any time without it affecting their medical care or relationship with the staff.

The committee will give particular attention to research involving patients who are unable by reason of age or mental disorder or intellectual disability to give informed consent and where such consent must be obtained from relatives or other responsible persons.

Where the design of the study is such that the researcher does not consider it necessary to seek fully informed consent from the research subjects, the committee must be satisfied with the reasons given for this conclusion, and with the extent to which information is withheld.

Scientific merit versus risks and costs to subjects

No study can be accepted as ethical unless the importance of the objective is in proportion to the inherent risks or other costs to the research subject.

The Committee will require to be satisfied on the clarity of the aims of the study and the statistical methods and power. Unless a study is likely to produce clinically or scientifically useful knowledge it cannot be considered ethical.

Competence of the investigators and adequacy of their facilities

The competence of the investigators to perform the study and the availability of adequate facilities must be established.

Confidentiality and security of data

Arrangements for confidentiality and security of data are required to comply with current guidelines, codes of practice and policy and, in the case of patient identifiable data held on computer and some manual records, with the statutory requirements of the Data Protection Act.

Informing medical attendants

The research subject's family doctor and/or consultant or other health professional in charge of their medical care must be informed of their participation in the study.

Mode of operation

► The committee shall meet at least once in every month.

► The committee shall consider every correctly completed application which it receives at its next available meeting provided that the application is received at least 10 working days prior to such a meeting.

► All completed applications and associated documents received by the secretary should be circulated with an agenda to all members, to be received by them at least five working days prior to the next meeting.

► The business of the committee shall be conducted in private to preserve confidentiality. A list of members present at the meeting will be provided on request, but *not* details of how individuals voted.

► If any member of the committee should have an interest of any kind in any research project, that member must leave the room while it is being considered and not participate in the decision.

► The committee will normally decide by consensus. Where this is not possible, it should be decided by a two-thirds majority of those present and any significant minority view recorded in the minutes.

► The committee will communicate its decisions to applicants with the minimum of delay and normally by letter within ten working days of the monthly meeting. The response should be helpful and, in (ii) to (iv) below, explain the reasons for the decision.

► The committee may: (i) formally approve a study; (ii) approve it conditional on certain points being addressed; (iii) defer it for consideration to a later meeting, to allow time for more information to be obtained from the researcher or for the researcher to attend the meeting; (iv) reject it.

► The committee may investigate the competence or qualifications of anyone involved in a research project or inspect the facilities involved.

► The committee will provide investigators with guidance on the information it requires to satisfy itself on the ethical acceptability of a study. A member of the committee, who is a clinician, may be identified as a source of informal advice to applicants.

► The committee may seek advice from outside its membership

when special expertise (medical or non-medical), not available within its membership, is required. To facilitate the consideration of particular applications, the committee may invite an appropriate expert to attend. Such persons must provide an undertaking of confidentiality and will not be entitled to vote on any matter.

▶ The committee may establish a small panel of assessors to consider non-routine submissions in depth and to make recommendations.

▶ The mode of operation of the committee shall be a matter for the chairperson and the committee to decide. The committee shall make a report to the health authority describing its method of operation and, in particular, its policy on unanimity and frequency of meetings.

Chairperson's action

▶ When a study is given conditional approval by the committee, once the required conditions have been adequately addressed by the researchers, it may be approved by chairperson's action without being referred back to the full committee.

▶ Minor protocol amendments not affecting patients may be approved by chairperson's action.

▶ The committee may agree that chairperson's action can be taken to approve certain kinds of study not involving invasive procedures or major ethical issues. When it is used for this purpose, the chairperson's decision must later be ratified by the full committee.

Post-approval responsibilities

▶ All amendments to the approved protocol affecting patients must be submitted to, and approved by, the committee before being implemented.

▶ The committee must be notified of all serious adverse events affecting patients in the trial whether locally or in other centres.

▶ In order to satisfy itself that medical research studies are being conducted in accordance with the proposal forms, protocol, information sheets and consent forms which have been approved, the committee reserves the right to conduct on-site monitoring of a sample of projects. Two committee members, or persons appointed by the committee, one of whom should be lay and the other medically qualified will perform the monitoring. The views of patients and volunteers regarding their participation in the research may also be canvassed.

▶ A monitoring meeting will include review of the following:

(i) identification of any difficulties in recruitment;

(ii) any changes to the approved protocol;

(iii) experience of adverse events;

(iv) the method of providing participants with information about the project and of obtaining consent;

(v) any refusal by a patient or volunteer to take part in the study;

(vi) any withdrawal from the study;

(vii) whether or not a final report is or will be available;

(viii) the number of consent forms available and the correctness of their completion;

(ix) the number of case record forms available and whether or not satisfactorily completed.

Committee records

The secretary shall:

▶ Prepare and maintain minutes of the meetings of the committee.

▶ Retain a copy of all applications and associated correspondence for at least 15 years.

▶ Keep a simple register of all applications made to the Committee, including the title of the project and the researcher's name and address.

Annual report

The committee shall submit an annual report to the health authority on its activities during the preceding year, which will be available for public inspection. It should list the proposals considered (taking care not to breach commercial confidentiality) and indicate the number approved. It should include a list of members serving on the committee. In its report, the committee may also draw attention to any matters deserving further attention or action by the authority, the university or any other body, and offer information and advice to researchers.

► Appendix 3
Specimen medical research ethics committee application form

The specimen proposal form given here is based on that currently used by the Tayside Committee on Medical Research Ethics which I revised with the help of committee members. The questions are designed to elicit the information about research projects that the committee needs in order to assess the ethical implications.

The committee also accepts multicentre applications on the standard form devised for use by the multicentre research ethics committees recently set up in the UK. The design of the national form, however, reflects the preponderance of pharmaceutical company sponsored trials that go to the multicentre committees. As these constitute only about 25 per cent of the workload of local committees, most committees still prefer to use a local form designed with a broader range of studies in mind, of which the one below is, I hope, a good example.

To reduce the amount of paper consumed and the need for expensive filing space, as access to personal computers increases, it should eventually become possible for ethics committees to accept proposals on electronic media.

(NAME) COMMITTEE ON MEDICAL RESEARCH ETHICS
PROPOSAL FOR CLINICAL RESEARCH

A copy of the form is available from the ethics committee on floppy disc in Microsoft Word for Windows version 6.0 and at the committee's Web site address.

Please note that research which is being conducted in five or more local ethics committee areas in the UK should be submitted initially to the appropriate multicentre research ethics committee.

(1) Title of proposed project: (as on grant application or protocol)

....

....

....

(2) Details of the researchers

(A) The researcher(s) responsible for the day to day management of the project.

► *(a) Principal researcher*

Name: ....

Qualifications: ....

Status: ....

Department: ....

Institute: ....

Address: ....

....

Telephone no. .... Extension ....

Bleep no. .... Fax no. .... E-mail ....

Name and address of employer: ....

....

....

....

For the researcher above, please state:

* How many years he/she has been involved in clinical research. ...
* The reference number of the last three submissions to the Ethics Committee and their status (for example, not initiated, in progress, completed and published). ....

....

....

....

▶ *(b) Second researcher*

Name: ....

Qualifications: ....

Status: ....

Department: ....

Institute: ....

Address: ....

....

Telephone no. .... Extension ....

Bleep no. .... Fax no. .... E-mail ....

Name and address of employer: ....

....

....

....

For the researcher above, please state:

• How many years he/she has been involved in clinical research. ...

• The reference number of the last three submissions to the Ethics Committee and their status (for example, not initiated, in progress, completed and published). ....

....

....

Extend the list if necessary

If the principal researcher is not medically qualified, please identify below who is providing medical cover. If this is not considered appropriate please explain.

(B) *Senior clinician (consultant or family doctor) with responsibility for the research.*

Name: ....

Qualifications: ....

Status: ....

Department: ....

Institute: ....

Address: ....

....

Telephone no. .... Extension ....

Bleep no. .... Fax no. .... E-mail ....

Name and address of employer: ....
....
....
....
....

(C) *If subjects are patients, the clinician(s) responsible for their care.*

Name: ....
Qualifications: ....
Status: ....
Department: ....
Institute: ....
Address: ....
....

Telephone no. .... Extension ....

    Bleep no. .... Fax no. .... E-mail ....

If the clinician is not a co-applicant has he/she seen and approved the proposal? (PLEASE TICK OR DELETE COMPLETELY.)

- • Yes ....
- • No ....

Extend the list if necessary

(D) *Who completed this form?*

Name: ....
If not included in the response to questions (2) or (3), please provide the details below:
Qualifications: ....
Status: ....
Department: ....
Institute: ....
Address: ....
....

Telephone no. .... Extension ....

    Bleep no. .... Fax no. .... E-mail ....

(Note: however responsibility for completing this form may be delegated, the researchers and other signatories are considered answerable by the ethics committee for what it contains.)

(E) *Who locally should be contacted about the project*

   • In non-urgent matters? ....
   ....

   • In an emergency? ....
   ....

(3) Sponsor/source of funding/financial matters

▶ *Who is sponsoring the study?*
   Contact name: ....
   Organisation: ....
   Address: ....
   ....

   • What is the level of payment? ....
   • Into what fund will the payment be credited and for what
      purpose is the fund to be used? ....
      ....

   • What undertaking has the researcher made as the basis for the
      payment (e.g. minimum number of patients to be recruited
      etc.)? ....
      ....

   • Give details of any provision of staff or equipment by the
      sponsor. ....
      ....

▶ *If no present sponsors, to whom has a grant application been, or is to
   be, made, or what is the source of the funding?* ....
   ....

▶ *Are any payments to be made to participants?*
   • Yes ....
   • No ....
      If yes, state the value and purpose of such payments (e.g.,
         travelling expenses). ....
      ....

▶ *Are the investigators free to publish the results of their findings?*
   • Yes ....
   • No ....

(4) Classification of the research

Please identify the type of research project involved. Tick as many items as necessary. (PLEASE TICK THOSE WHICH APPLY OR DELETE THOSE WHICH DO NOT.)

▶ *The type of participant: – **Remember to include those to be used as controls.***
- Healthy volunteers ....
- Family doctor patients ....
- Outpatients ....
- Inpatients ....
- Other (please specify) ....

▶ *The scale of the study:*
- Single centre ....
- National multicentre (under five centres) ....
- National multicentre (five or more centres) ....
- International multicentre ....

▶ *The type of research:*
(a) Commercially sponsored research
- Sponsor-initiated contract research for drug development with sponsor's protocol ....
- Sponsored research for drug development but with local protocol ....
- Other product or equipment development ....
(b) Academic, health services, government and non-commercial research
- Basic clinical research with patients ....
- Basic clinical research involving spare blood samples etc. ....
- Cost effectiveness ....
- Diagnostic imaging ....
- Embryo research ....
- Epidemiological survey ....
- Equipment ....
- Genetic screening ....
- Health Promotion ....
- Measurement/Test/Assay ....

- Nutrition ....
- Patient satisfaction ....
- Provision of services ....
- Research including questionnaires ....
- Research involving questionnaires *only* ....
- Research involving access to medical records with no patient contact ....
- Social survey ....
- Surgical procedures ....
- Others (please specify) ....

► *Purpose of study:*
- Satisfying drug development regulations ....
- To further understanding of a condition and its treatment. ....
- Undergraduate/postgraduate project ....
- Other (please specify) ....
  ....

(5) The protocol

► *Is there a pre-existing protocol for this study?*
- Yes ....
- No ....
  If yes, have you submitted a copy with this application?
  - Yes ....
  - No ....
  If no, this form will be considered as the protocol for the study by the ethics committee.

(6) Previous assessment

► *Has the research been approved by any other Research Ethics Committee?*
- Yes ....
- No ....
  If yes, please give details. ....
  ....
  ....

► *Has the proposal to your knowledge been turned down by another Research Ethics Committee?*
  - Yes ....
  - No ....
    If yes, please give the reasons. ....
    ....
    ....

► *If similar research has been approved by this Committee before, please give our reference numbers:* ....
    ....

► *Has the project been peer-reviewed?*
  - Yes ....
  - No ....
    If yes, who by and what was the outcome?...................................
    ....

► *What kind of literature review has been carried out to see whether this or similar research has been done before?* ....
    ....

(7) Starting dates and duration
Please state:
  - The likely starting date of the project in this centre and the likely total duration of the collection of the clinical/biomedical data. ....
    ....
  - The likely starting date for participants, and the duration for which *each individual participant* will be in the study. ....
    ....
  - The premises in which the project will be undertaken. ....
    ....

(8) Details of the research project
  - The local researchers should give their own summary (about one page i.e. 210 x 297 mm, 8.27 x 11.69 in) of the proposed project in language comprehensible to both medical and lay

members of the committee. This should cover the background and justification for this research and what it will actually involve for patients.

....

....

....

....

....

....

....

....

....

....

....

....

....

....

- Is the power of the study sufficient to answer the question that is being asked? Who did the statistical calculation and where is it recorded? (Note: if this is a pilot study, say so.)

....

(9) The participants

Please give the following information in respect of the patients and controls or healthy volunteers taking part in the research.

▶ *Who are the proposed participants (including controls if appropriate)?* ....

....

▶ *How are they to be selected?*
- What inclusion criteria will be used? ....
- What exclusion criteria will be used? ....

....

▶ *Age range* ....

▶ *Sex* ....

► *Numbers involved:*
  • In this centre   Patients: ....
                     Controls/healthy volunteers: ....
  • Overall   Patients: ....
                     Controls/healthy volunteers: ....

► *Please state if any of the participants are:*
  • Students or staff of the researchers
    Yes ....
    No ....
  • Patients of the researchers
    Yes ....
    No ....
  • Patients of the consultant in charge of the study
    Yes ....
    No ....
  • Patients in the same department as the researchers
    Yes ....
    No ....
  • Other relationship (please specify) ....

► *Are any participants likely to be involved in existing research, or to have been involved in any research within the last three months?*
  • Yes ....
  • No ....
    If yes, please justify their participation in this project. ....
    ....

(10) Obtaining informed consent

A PATIENT/VOLUNTEER INFORMATION SHEET WRITTEN IN PLAIN, NON-TECHNICAL LANGUAGE MUST BE ATTACHED TO THIS PROPOSAL FORM.

SEE THE COMMITTEE'S "GUIDE TO CONSTRUCTING A PATIENT/ VOLUNTEER INFORMATION SHEET."

► *If written consent is not to be obtained, please justify.* ....
....

- ▶ *Will the Medical Research Ethics Committee's standard consent form be used?*
  - • Yes ....
  - • No ....

    If no, please give the reason and attach the form you wish to use.

- ▶ *Who will seek consent from the potential participant/carer?* ....

- ▶ *Describe how and when potential participants will be approached with information about the project.* ....
  ....

- ▶ *How long will the potential participants have to decide whether to take part in the study before being asked to sign the consent form? If less than 24 hours, please justify.* ....
  ....

- ▶ *Are any participants in the study likely to have problems in giving informed consent?*
  - • Yes ....
  - • No ....

    If yes, explain the reason (e.g., age, mental illness, dementia, communication difficulties, unconsciousness, or other reasons?)
    ....
    ....

    If yes, what special arrangements have been made to deal with the issue of consent?
    ....
    ....

- ▶ *What special arrangements have been made for participants whose first language is not English?* ....
  ....
  ....

(11) The influence of the research on the normal treatment of patients

▶ *In cases of therapeutic research involving patients, describe the alternative/standard treatments (if any), which they would normally receive in the absence of the research.* ....

....

....

▶ *Are patients on long-term medication for their condition which is to be discontinued for purposes of this study, or is standard treatment to be withheld from newly diagnosed patients?*

- Yes ....
- No ....

If yes, state:

- what is the ethical justification for withholding the established medication. ....

....

- what percentage of the patients recruited will be on placebo medication and for how long (e.g. 100% for washout period of four weeks plus 33% for one year). ....

....

- what rescue medication will be available and the criteria under which the patients themselves or the researchers will use it. ....

....

▶ *What are the plans for treating patients at the end of the formal trial? If the drug proves beneficial to them, is the sponsor able to make it available to them or will they revert to previous or standard medication?* ....

....

▶ *Are there are any expected benefits to:*
(a) Participants including any control or placebo group?

- Yes ....
- No ....

If yes, please describe what they are. ....

....

(b) Future patients?

- Yes ....
- No ....

  If yes, please describe what they are. ....

  ....

(12) Hazards and discomforts

▶ *Please list those procedures in the study to which participants will be exposed. Indicate those which would be part of normal care and those which will be additional (e.g., a qualifying diagnostic test or taking more samples than would otherwise be necessary).* ....

....

....

If there are any *additional* procedures, describe any associated hazards and give their anticipated frequency and morbidity. ....

....

....

▶ *Does the research involve the* WITHHOLDING *of standard investigations or treatments?*

- Yes ....
- No ....

  If yes, describe any associated hazards and give their anticipated frequency and morbidity. ....

  ....

  ....

  ....

▶ *Are there any other potential hazards to participants arising from the research?*

- Yes ....
- No ....

  If yes, what is the anticipated frequency and morbidity of these hazards and what precautions are to be taken to meet them?

  ....

  ....

▶ *Are there any procedures in the research project which may cause discomfort or distress to participants?*
- Yes ....
- No ....
  If yes, describe the degree of discomfort or distress entailed and their estimated probability. ....
  ....
  ....

  Is there any alternative to these procedures? If so please describe. ...
  ....
  ....

▶ *Please describe any special withdrawal criteria (e.g. in a trial of a new antihypertensive, elevation of the patient's blood pressure above a certain level.)* ....
  ....
  ....

▶ **RADIATION HAZARDS.**
  (a) Will any ionising or radioactive substances or x-rays be administered?
- Yes ....
- No ....
  If yes, please give details of:
  - the radioactive substances to be administered (investigation, radionucleide, chemical form, ...
  - the quantity to be administered (MBq), route and frequency), ...
    ....
  - the Estimated Effective Dose(Effective Dose Equivalent) (mSv), ...
  - the absorbed dose to organ or tissue(specify) concentrating the radioactivity (mGy), ...
  and/or
  - details of radiographic procedures (investigation, organ and frequency) ....
    ....

* the Estimated Effective Dose(Effective Dose Equivalent)
   (mSv). ....
   ....

(b) Has an application been made to the Area Radiation Safety
Committee?
* Yes ....
* No ....
(c) Date of application: ....

(13) The drugs involved

▶ *Does the research application concern a new (non formulary)
   medicinal product or new medical device?*
   * Yes ....
   * No ....

▶ *Does the research application concern the novel use of an approved
   product outside the terms of the product licence?*
   * Yes ....
   * No ....

▶ *For ALL drugs employed, whether non-formulary or marketed, give:*
   * The generic or code names, strengths, dosage and frequency,
     and route of administration: ....
     ....
     ....
   * a summary of known toxic effects on humans: ....
     ....
     ....

▶ *Is a Clinical Trial Exemption Certificate required for this study?*
   * Yes ....
   * No ....
     If yes, has a Clinical Trial Exemption Certificate been obtained
        from the Committee on Safety of Medicines?
     * Yes ....
     * No ....

(14) Confidentiality

► *Please state who will have access to the data.* ....
....

► *Will it be possible to link any results obtained to individual participants?*
  - Yes ....
  - No ....

    If yes, state whether any results of significance to the participants will be communicated to them or to their family doctors. ....

► *What steps will be taken to safeguard the confidentiality of:*
  - personal record? ....
    ....
  - personal laboratory specimens? ....
    ....
  - audio or video recordings? ....
    ....

► *If the study data is to be held on, or retrieved from, computer will the requirements of the Data Protection Act (1984) be adhered to?* ....

(15) Insurance

► *Have arrangements been made to provide indemnification and/or compensation in the event of a claim by, or on behalf of, a subject for:*
  (a) negligent harm?
  - Yes ....
  - No ....
  - Not applicable ....

    If yes, please give details and provide a copy of the indemnity form with this application. If no, or not applicable, please explain. ....
    ....
    ....

  (b) non-negligent harm?
  (For pharmaceutical company sponsored research in the UK, the company should conform to the most recent Association of British Pharmaceutical Industrys' guidelines.)

- Yes ....
- No ....
- Not applicable ....
  If yes, please give details. If no, or not applicable, please explain.

  ....

  ....

▶ *In cases of equipment or medical devices, have appropriate*
  arrangements been made with the manufacturer to provide
  indemnification?
  - Yes ....
  - No ....
  - Not applicable ....
    If yes, please give details. If no, or not applicable, please explain.

    ....

    ....

(16) Consulting with family doctors

▶ *If the study involves **healthy volunteers**, will you seek the advice of*
  the family doctor concerning their suitability to participate, and any
  health risks involved?
  - Yes ....
  - No ....
    If yes, please enclose a copy of the letter.

▶ *If the study involves **patients**, do you intend to inform their family*
  doctor, or other health professional normally in charge of their care,
  of their participation?
  - Yes ....
  - No ....
    If yes, please enclose a copy of the letter.

▶ *Does the study involve the active participation of the family doctor*
  or other member(s) of the primary care team?
  - Yes ....
  - No ....
    If yes, have you obtained the family doctor's support?
    - Yes ....
    - No ....

(17) Additional ethical considerations

► *What particular ethical issues do you think are raised by the proposed study?*..

....

....

(18) Final check

► *Other relevant material*
  Have you enclosed the following?
  (a) All participant/carer information sheets   Yes......No......N A......
  (b) The Company Protocol and Investigator's
       Brochure (one copy only)   Yes......No......N A......
  (c) Letters to participants   Yes......No......N A......
  (d) Copies of advertisements or any other
       recruiting material   Yes......No......N A......
  (e) Letters to family doctors   Yes......No......N A......
  (f) Questionnaires   Yes......No......N A......
  (g) Others, please specify   Yes......No......N A......
  (h) The signed declarations   Yes......No......N A......

(*NUMBER*) *COLLATED* COPIES OF THE PROPOSAL FORM, PARTICIPANT INFORMATION SHEETS AND OTHER RELEVANT ENCLOSURES SHOULD BE SUBMITTED.

(To save paper and filing space, it is preferable to print on both sides of the paper.)

For commercially sponsored studies where the information to be obtained is for the benefit of the company, a fee will be charged for the review of applications. This is currently (*amount*), an invoice for which will be raised by the Finance Department.

Please submit the application form to:
(*Name*)
Secretary,
(*Name*) Committee on Medical Research Ethics,
(*Name*) Organisation,
(*Address*)

Telephone No.   Extension
Fax No.
E-mail

(19) Declaration

Principal researcher

I confirm that this document is an accurate and complete account of the intended research, that I have read it thoroughly, and that it has my approval and commitment.

   I will ensure that any changes to the protocol are submitted to the ethics committee for approval prior to their implementation, and that serious adverse reactions will be notified to the committee with the minimum of delay.

The research will be conducted in accordance with the principles of the Declaration of Helsinki and its Amendments.

I confirm that I am familiar with these principles.

Signed ....

(NAME IN CAPITALS) ....

Date ....

Second researcher

I confirm that this document is an accurate and complete account of the intended research, that I have read it thoroughly, and that it has my approval and commitment.

   I will ensure that any changes to the protocol are submitted to the ethics committee for approval prior to their implementation, and that serious adverse reactions will be notified to the committee with the minimum of delay.

The research will be conducted in accordance with the principles of the Declaration of Helsinki and its Amendments.

I confirm that I am familiar with these principles.

Signed ....

(NAME IN CAPITALS) ....

Date ....

Senior clinician with responsibility for the research

This will normally be the responsible clinical consultant where the applicant is not of that grade (unless the researcher is a family doctor).

I confirm that I am answerable for the clinical conduct of this research, that I have read and checked this proposal and consider the answers to be appropriate and reasonable.

I confirm that those conducting the research are adequately experienced in the research procedures and in the medical ethics and that the research will be conducted in accordance with the principles of the Declaration of Helsinki and its Amendments.

Signed ....

(NAME IN CAPITALS) ....

Date ....

(Or) *Consultant, not having responsibility for the research, but for the clinical care of the patients involved.*

I confirm that I have clinical responsibility for patients involved in this research; that the researchers have introduced themselves and have acquainted me with the nature of their research; and that I have approved both the project and the researchers.

Signed ....

(NAME IN CAPITALS) ....

Date ....

► Appendix 4
Guide to constructing a patient/volunteer information sheet

The information sheet should contain the full title of the proposal except where this might be disturbing to patients. Care should be taken in the choice of words for the title. It may for instance be inappropriate to use the word 'cancer' in sheets intended for cancer patients at home. Many patients, having been informed of the diagnosis, use denial as a coping mechanism, and choose to avoid the knowledge that they have a life limiting illness. Using the word 'cancer' in the information sheet, in some cases might be an insensitive way of reintroducing bad news that the patient has chosen to forget, ignore, or bury in their subconscious.

When the title is not self-explanatory, the meaning of technical terms such as 'cross-over study' or 'double blind' should be explained. A simpler title may be used *in addition* to the formal title, care being taken to ensure that it is not persuasive.

Information Sheets for healthy volunteers should be clearly labelled *Healthy Volunteer Information Sheet*.

The information sheet should begin with an invitation to participate:

> We invite you to participate in a research project. We believe it to be of potential importance. However, before you decide whether or not you wish to participate, we need to be sure that you understand, firstly why we are doing it and, secondly what it would involve if you agreed. We are therefore providing you with the following information. Read it carefully and be sure to ask any questions you have and, if you wish, discuss it with relatives,

friends or anyone else. We will do our best to explain and to provide any further information you may ask for now or later. You do not have to make an immediate decision.

The Information Sheet should then provide answers to as many of the following questions as are relevant to the study, care being taken to explain the study in language which is neither too patronising nor too technically complex.

I have used section headings corresponding to the eight basic elements of informed consent required by the American regulations (45 CFR, 46.11a; 21 CFR, 50.25a) as this provides a convenient layout for the information sheet while equally satisfying the UK (Royal College of Physicians 1986b, 1990a,b, s.7.14) requirements and the international requirements for pharmaceutical trials (International Conference on Harmonisation 1996, s.4.8.10). The individual questions are mine. The bracketed letter after certain questions indicates that the question accords with one of the 20 items of information required to be given to patients by the International Conference of Harmonisation (ICH) guideline (ICH 1996, s.4.8.10 a–t)

- **A statement that research is being conducted, its purposes, duration, and a description of the experimental procedures to be employed**
  - ► What is the research about? *(a)*
  - ► What is the purpose of the research ? *(b)*
  - ► Who is sponsoring it, and are they paying the researcher or the department to do the research?
  - ► Why have I been chosen as a possible participant in the research?
  - ► How long will my participation in the study last? *(s)*
  - ► Will I have to come back to the clinic more often, or remain in hospital longer, than would normally be the case? *(f)*
  - ► What are my responsibilities? *(e)*
  - ► What procedures will I be asked to submit to and what will they be like? *(d)*

► What treatment will I get if I do take part?
► Will the decisions about my treatment be made by my usual doctor or by someone else?
► Will the treatment be decided at random? *(c)*
► What are the names and amounts of the drugs that I will be given (if any) and by what route?
► Will all patients receive active treatment, or will some receive dummy medication? If so, what is the chance that I would receive dummy medication?

● ● ● Description of foreseeable risks and side-effects to the subject *(g)*

► Are there any factors that would exclude me from participating, such as pre-existing illness, the possibility of becoming pregnant, or other drugs being taken?
► Will there be any discomforts, such as additional needle pricks or biopsies, or pain, and if so, how much and for how long?
► Are there likely to be side effects from what will be done to me in the research, and if so what are they?
► Were I to feel severe discomfort or pain during the study would I be able to take any relief medication?
► Is there any chance of anything going wrong, and if so, what?
► What are the risks of anything going wrong compared to everyday activities?
► Are there any activities I should refrain from during, and in the period following, the research and for how long, for example, blood donations, taking other medication, exposure to sunlight, driving, taking part in other studies?

How much information about risks and benefits should the patient be given?

In standard clinical practice in the UK, full disclosure of all of the risks and benefits of a procedure is generally not considered to be necessary for consent to be valid, doctors having only to reveal as much information as would be revealed by any responsible and skilled body of their peers. It must be acknowledged, however, that not everyone would consider this level of information to be acceptable. With research procedures, as the intention may not be to directly benefit the participants, more complete disclosure of risks is necessary than is the case where patients are receiving treatments likely to be of direct benefit to them.

Where they are known, all of the significant potential risks and side-effects should be given, with some indication of their frequency in everyday terms. Where a new drug is being tested, the side-effects of the standard treatment should be given for comparison. The extent to which risks should be revealed is discussed in more detail in Chapter 5.

A description of benefits to subjects or to others *(h)*

▶ Is there any chance that the proposed research will be of benefit to me personally, or to future patients with the same condition?

▶ If so, what are the potential benefits?

▶ Were the new treatment to be of benefit to me, could I continue to take it after the trial?

▶ If not, what medical care and follow-up will I receive after the trial?

Description of alternative treatments available

▶ What treatment will I get if I do not take part? *(i)*

▶ How will the treatment that I will get, and the procedures to which I will be exposed, if I do take part differ from the standard treatment and procedures? *(f)*

Statement regarding confidentiality

▶ How will my confidentiality be protected, i.e. who will have access to the records generated and what steps will be taken to ensure that they will only be seen by those authorised to see them? *(n)* (Remember to include the possibility of audit by drug company or regulatory agency representatives where appropriate, or post-approval review by the ethics committee.)

► Will my family doctor be told that I am taking part in this study, and the results of my participation?

► If any illness of which I am presently unaware is found as a result of the study, will I be told and receive any treatment for it?

► If the research may result in me or my relatives being made aware for the first time of our susceptibility to an illness, what arrangements have been made for counselling?

► Will I be informed of the results of the study?

► Will I be identified in any publications arising from the research? *(o)*

●●● Arrangements for compensation should the subject be harmed *(j)*

► If something went wrong, how and from whom would I obtain compensation? (If the study is sponsored by an industrial company, the specific arrangements such as, in the UK, an agreement to abide by Association of the British Pharmaceutical Industry guidelines should be specified.)

●●● Who should be contacted for further information or in the event of injury *(q)*

► How can I obtain more information if I wish?

► Who would I be able to contact if I became worried about any side-effects that I experienced?

► Who would I need to contact in order to claim compensation?

●●● Statement that participation is voluntary *(m)*

► Can I discuss the study with friends and relatives, or my family doctor before deciding whether or not to take part?

► Can I refuse to take part or change my mind later even if I agree to take part now?

► If I do refuse to take part or change my mind later, will I still get the treatment my usual doctor thinks is right for me?

The information sheet should contain the following statement or a near equivalent regarding the voluntary nature of participation:

We stress that participation in this study is entirely voluntary. You are free to decline to take part and you can withdraw from the study at any time without having to give a reason. This would not affect your present or future medical care or your relationship with the staff looking after you.

Additional elements of informed consent

► Is it possible that there may be unforeseeable risks to myself (or to the embryo or fetus if I become pregnant)?

► In what circumstances might the investigator terminate my participation without my consent? *(r)*

► May I incur any additional costs as a result of participation (e.g. will I get travelling or other expenses or other payment)? *(k, l)*

► What would be the consequences of my decision to withdraw and what would be the procedures for orderly termination of my participation?

► Does the researcher agree to provide me with relevant information arising during the course of the trial which may influence my decision whether or not to continue to participate? *(p)*

► How many other participants will be involved in the study (i.e. in this centre and overall)? *(t)*

Ensure that copies of the Information Sheet are available for all who might need them

Include a copy of the information sheet (and consent form) in the patient's hospital case notes, so that other doctors who might be involved in their treatment for the same, or an unrelated, condition are aware of their participation in a trial and can contact the researcher if there are any fears about drug or other interactions. Keep the original consent form with the research records securely under lock and key.

Allow the patient/volunteer adequate time to decide whether to participate

The patient/volunteer should, whenever the nature of the study allows, be given several days to discuss the information sheet with friends and relatives or their family doctor before deciding whether to participate. Those who decide to participate should then be given the standard (*name*) Medical Research Ethics Committee Consent Form, or an approved alternative, to sign.

Pitfalls to avoid in writing information leaflets

Avoid alarming patients unnecessarily

In one study of heart disease the patient was told: 'This extra strain on the heart is thought to predispose people like yourself to further heart attacks, further damage to your heart or even death'. This may be true but need it be put quite so bluntly? The ethics committee asked the researcher to try and be more tactful. The following sentence of the same information sheet read: 'We have a new drug which opposes the action of this damaging hormone'. Persuasion too, as who would not now want to receive the drug, seeing it as their only hope of survival!

The careless use of medical terminology can also alarm patients. A patient information sheet may begin: 'Your doctor will have told you that you have heart failure.' The term 'heart failure' has alarming connotations, which are not always justified, as there are varying degrees of this condition. How much nicer to say, 'Your doctor will have told you that you are suffering from cardiac insufficiency, sometimes referred to as heart failure, which means that your heart is not pumping as well as it could be and this is why you are taking medication'.

Using expressions such as 'surrogates of mortality', although a useful and widely used concept for researchers, will be totally meaningless to the vast majority of participants, and may even conjure up terrifying images for some people. These should therefore be avoided as should using statements that could cause offence, for example 'couples like you who are infertile'.

Ensure that control subjects are given the correct information sheet

Information sheets should be clearly labelled either *Patient Information Sheet*, or *Healthy Volunteer Information Sheet* to show who they are intended for. Otherwise, it is all too easy for the person seeking consent to inadvertently hand a patient information sheet to a healthy control. This is especially important when patients in hospital for a condition unrelated to the illness being studied are selected as controls. Given the wrong information sheet, they may imagine that they have been diagnosed with an illness which no one has previously told them about.

Consideration should also be given to what may happen to information sheets after they leave the hospital. An unambiguous *Healthy Volunteer* heading in large print will reduce the possibility of an acquaintance of the volunteer getting the mistaken impression from a casual glance at an information sheet left carelessly lying about that the volunteer is suffering from a serious illness. A simple precaution such as providing the information sheet in an envelope may also reduce the number of breaches of confidentiality that occur in patients' own homes.

Avoid silly acronyms

There is a tendency for some investigators, especially sponsors of multi-centre trials, to give their studies heroic sounding acronyms. These can be irritating both to ethics committees and to patients, particularly if the title of the study has obviously been contrived to fit the acronym rather than the other way round, rendering the title contorted and incomprehensible. In the worst cases, acronyms can be offensive, by appearing to trivialise a serious condition, or with a title like SUCCESS (Study to Understand Cancer Chemotherapy Effectiveness in Seven Sites), by implying that the benefits are more probable than they really are.

Avoid unnecessary technical jargon

The information sheet should be written in simple, but not patronising, non-technical language that the patient can readily understand. In writing patient information sheets, many researchers seem to imagine that patients are specialists in their area of research and use so much in-house jargon that even medical members of research ethics committees have difficulty in understanding what the study is about. On the other hand, some patient groups, such as those with asthma, diabetes or haemophilia, are often extremely well informed about their condition and can take the jargon in their stride.

Abbreviations are a major obstacle to communicating meaning, as they may mean different things to different people, and should be avoided as far as possible. Take DNA. To a geneticist it means the genetic material, deoxyribonucleic acid, but to an outpatient records officer it means Did Not Attend. To most people such abbreviations usually mean nothing at all.

The author of the information sheet should try it out first on non-medical friends or relatives before presenting it to patients. The ability to communicate effectively with patients is an essential qualification for medical practitioners, and a readily comprehensible information sheet is therefore to be expected.

Avoid coercive language

The use of persuasive language is extremely common in information sheets arising no doubt as an innocent result of the researchers' enthusiasm for their research. 'We hope that you will agree to join the study'; 'We would be grateful if you would agree to be interviewed'; 'We would be grateful if you would allow us to . . .'; 'You are not obliged to participate, but we very much hope you will'. Expressions such as these should be avoided.

Neither should patient information sheets be worded as though the patient is definitely going to participate. This effect can be produced by the researcher launching into a description of what *will* happen to the patient: 'You *will* take this tablet'; 'You *will* give this sample', etc. Such statements should always be prefaced by the condition: 'If you agree to participate'.

The voluntary nature of participation and the right to withdraw at any time should always be emphasised in the information sheet. Patients not wishing to participate in a study should never be challenged as to why they do not wish to do so.

Avoid bad grammar and spelling mistakes

A patient information sheet written with poor grammar and full of spelling errors gives a bad impression to patients and members of the ethics committee. It has to be remembered that although the project as a whole may be brilliantly conceived, all patients usually see of it is the Information Sheet. Many people associate the ability to spell with a good education, and may even distrust an English speaking doctor who cannot spell properly in English or who does not know the difference between the meaning of words such as 'affect' and 'effect' or 'their' and 'there'.

As all current word processing software includes a spell checker, there is little excuse for presenting patients with non-existent words. (I hope there are not too many in this book!) It is also advisable to have another person who is not directly involved with the research to read through the information sheet to make sure there are no obvious spelling mistakes and that the sense is clear. Poor grammar frequently arises in international multi-centre trials owing to the patient information sheet having been poorly translated from one language into another. Local researchers should check translated information sheets carefully and re-phrase them as necessary before submitting them to the ethics committee.

Can the patient read it?

Even a well written information sheet is of limited value if patients are unable to read it. As many patients are older people with a significant possibility of failing eye sight, the print size used in a patient information sheet should always reflect this. It is also unwise to assume that everyone can read English (or other relevant language). If it is intended to recruit participants whose native language is not English, the text should be appropriately translated. For those who are unable to read any language effectively, for example because of poor eyesight or education, serious consideration should be given to providing the information on audiotape. This should be done in addition to a live verbal explanation, as a tape, like a paper sheet, has the advantage that it can be 'read' over and over again until the patient gets a feel for what is going on and eventually understands enough about it at least to appreciate what is not understood so that questions can be asked. In such cases care must be taken not to insult the intelligence of the patient by using over-simplified language.

Presentation is important. A page of unbroken text can be extremely tedious to read. It is much better to break it up with suitable headings such as:

- ► Background to the research and its aims.
- ► What is involved for participants.
- ► Risks and side-effects.
- ► Potential benefits.
- ► Alternative treatments available.
- ► Confidentiality.
- ► Arrangements for compensation.
- ► To obtain further information.
- ► Participation is entirely voluntary.

Sentence construction is also important. Beware of overlong sentences with more than one dependent clause. If a point is important, it deserves a sentence to itself.

Most modern word processing software includes a readability score. Run it to see whether what you have written is likely to be readable by its intended audience. Those of us who spend much of our lives reading and writing often fail to appreciate that for a significant proportion of the population, although they may be highly skilled in other areas, reading does not come easily.

Final check for grammar and spelling

Ensure that the information sheet is clearly presented in an appropriate type size, and is free of grammatical and spelling errors. It is important that the information sheet is clearly and logically laid out so that it appears 'friendly' and not overly 'formal' which can so easily put individuals off reading carefully through text.

As an aid to confidentiality, participants should be given an envelope marked 'CONFIDENTIAL' into which to put the information sheet when they take it home.

An information leaflet rather than an information sheet?

Rather than just providing sheets of paper, modern word processing software makes it easy to present the information in the form of a simple information leaflet, which looks more professional, and can often be exploited to break up the text more clearly into sections.

Don't ignore the verbal explanation

In the struggle to produce a well written information sheet, the importance of a clear verbal explanation should not be overlooked. The two are complementary. Some researchers can express themselves better verbally than in writing, while others are better at written than verbal communication. Similarly, while some patients may find the spoken word easier to comprehend than the written, others prefer to mull over the written word. Presenting information both verbally and as a written information sheet is likely to increase the level of the patient's understanding. When patients are unable to read for whatever reason, a clear verbal explanation is obviously vital.

► Appendix 5
A specimen consent form for patients

(This form can be modified for
carers or healthy volunteers)

(TITLE OF PROPOSAL)

Patient Consent Form

To be completed by the patient	Please cross out as necessary
Have you read the Patient Information Sheet?	Yes/No
Have you had an opportunity to ask questions and discuss this study?	Yes/No
Have you received satisfactory answers to all of your questions?	Yes/No
Have you received enough information about the study?	Yes/No
Who have you spoken to? Dr/Mr/Mrs/Miss	
Do you understand that participation is entirely voluntary?	Yes/No
Do you understand that you are free to withdraw from the study: • at any time? • without having to give a reason for withdrawing? • without this affecting your future medical care?	Yes/No
Do you agree to take part in this study?	Yes/No

► *Patient's signature*...*Date*...........................
Patient's name (in block letters) ....
Telephone number where patient can be contacted:
.... (Home)..(Work)

► *Doctor's signature*..*Date*...........................

The investigator should give a copy of the consent form and information sheet to the participant to keep, insert a copy in their clinical case notes; and keep the top copy in the research records for ease of access and checking by monitors from the regulatory authorities, drug company or ethics committee.

(a) The above form is based on that recommended by the Royal College of Physicians (1990b, s.7.20) with the addition of the question regarding the voluntary nature of participation, a space for the patient's telephone number and the doctor's signature.

(b) The production of multiple copies is made easier if consent forms are professionally printed on specially coated paper so that copies are automatically produced as the top copy is completed.

A specimen letter and confidential questionnaire for patients/healthy volunteers

LETTER

Dear

(Title of the study)
The aim of the enclosed questionnaire is to help us to improve our service to patients and volunteers involved in research. It has been designed by the *(Name)* Committee on Medical Research Ethics/ Institutional Review Board (IRB) to find out how people feel about their participation in research studies. The Committee/IRB will produce a report outlining the findings of the survey and make recommendations to help researchers to improve their service to participants.

Please return this questionnaire if you wish (there is of course no obligation to do so) in the pre-paid envelope provided (no stamp required) to *(Name)*, Secretary, *(Name)* Committee on Medical Research Ethics/IRB, *(Name)* Hospital, *(Address)*.

We would like to assure you that your comments will be completely confidential. They will not be seen by myself or other members of the research team, but only by members of the ethics committee.

Yours sincerely

Senior Researcher

CONFIDENTIAL QUESTIONNAIRE FOR PATIENTS/HEALTHY VOLUNTEERS

Study number

Study title

This questionnaire mainly consists of ticking answers, but please feel free to make any additional comments as you wish.

Section A

The questions in Section A ask about the information you were given to help you decide whether or not to take part in the study.

▶ *(A1) Were you given an Information Sheet when you were first asked to consider participating?*

        Yes ....   No ....

   • **If no, go to question (A6).**

   Did you read it?

        Yes ....   No ....

   • **If not, please give the reason, if you can remember, then go to question (A6).** ....

   ....

   ....

▶ *(A2) Was the Information Sheet easy or difficult to understand?*

   Easy to understand   ....

   Some parts were easy and some were difficult........

   Difficult to understand   ....

   If you can remember, please say which, if any, were the difficult parts? ....

   ....

   ....

▶ *(A3) Did the Information Sheet answer most of your questions?*

   All   ....

   Nearly all   ....

   Some questions unanswered   ....

   A lot of questions unanswered   ....

▶ *(A4) Was the Information Sheet:*

Too short ....
About the right length ....
Too long ....
Too patronising ....
Too technical ....

▶ *(A5) Did someone go through the information sheet with you, carefully explaining any difficult parts?*

Yes .... No ....

▶ *(A6) Who did you talk to about the study?*

Your doctor ....
Nurse ....
Another doctor ....
Other, please specify ....
Their name(s), if you know ....
....

No one
  • **If no one, go to question (A11).**

▶ *(A7) Did you have plenty of time to talk to him/her about the Study?*

Yes .... No ....

▶ *(A8) Did you find it easy to ask him/her questions?*

Yes .... No ....
If not, can you explain why not? ....
....

▶ *(A9) Did you understand his/her answers?*

Yes .... Some of them .... No ....

▶ *(A10) Which of the following did you find most helpful in understanding the study? (Tick one line)*

The Information Sheet ....
Talking to the researcher in charge of the
  study ....

Talking to other researchers, medical or nursing
    staff   ....
Talking to your hospital doctor   ....
Talking to your family doctor   ....
Talking to anyone else?   ....
    Please say who: ....

....

► *(A11) Can you write down briefly in a few sentences why the study was being carried out, as you understand it.*

....
....
....

Section B

The questions in Section B ask you whether your decision to participate was made freely.

► *(B1) Did you feel that you were under any pressure to take part in the study?*

    Yes ....   Some ....   No ....
  • **If no, go to question (B3).**

► *(B2) If yes, or some, from who or what did you feel the pressure was coming?*

Doctors   ....
Family members   ....
Researchers   ....
Nurses   ....
A feeling you should show gratitude   ....
A feeling that the medical staff might be
    upset if you didn't take part   ....
A feeling that you might not get so much
    attention if you didn't take part   ....
Other   ....
    Please explain: ....

....

▶ *(B3) Did you feel that anyone was putting any pressure on you* NOT
to join the study?

Yes .... Some .... No
• **If no, go to question (B5).**

▶ *(B4) If yes, or some, who was the pressure coming from?*

Doctor ....
Family members ....
Other ....
Please explain: ....
....

▶ *(B5) How long **were you given** to make your mind up about
whether to take part in the study?*

A few minutes ....
About an hour ....
A few hours ....
A day ....
A few days ....
A week or longer ....

▶ *(B6) How long **did you take** to make your mind up about whether to
take part in the study?*

A few minutes ....
About an hour ....
A few hours ....
A day ....
A few days ....
A week or longer ....

▶ *(B7) Do you feel you were given sufficient time to think about the
study or discuss it with your relatives or family doctor before
you had to decide whether or not to take part?*

Yes .... No ....
If no, can you please add any comments you
wish to make (such as when you think you
should have first been approached about it). .....
....

Section C

The questions in Section C ask about your experience of being in the study.

▶ *(C1) Since joining the study have any questions come to mind?*

Yes .... No ....
• **If no, go to question (C3).**

▶ *(C2) If yes, who did you ask?*

Doctor ....
Other ....
Family doctor ....
No one ....
If you had questions, but did not ask anyone,
please say what prevented you. ....
....

▶ *(C3) Have you experienced any difficulties in travelling or making domestic or working arrangements to take part in the study?*

Yes .... No ....
If yes, can you please explain. ....
....

▶ *(C4) Have you incurred any additional expense which you did not expect as a result of taking part in the study?*

Yes .... No ....
If yes, can you please explain. ....
....

▶ *(C5) Has anything happened to you in this study which has caused you, or continues to cause you, any concern?*

Yes .... No ....
If yes, can you please explain. ....
....

▶ *(C6) Have you been kept fully informed about what is happening at each stage in the study?*

Yes .... No ....

▶ *(C7) Now that you have taken part in this study, are you more, or less, likely to take part in another study in the future?*

    More likely   ....

    No change   ....

    Less likely   ....

    Definitely not   ....

    If more, or less likely, please explain why ....

    ....

    ....

▶ *(C8) Any additional comments you may wish to make about the study.*

    ....

    ....

    ....

    ....

    ....

    ....

    ....

    ....

► Appendix 7
A specimen review questionnaire for researchers

(*NAME*) RESEARCH ETHICS COMMITTEE/ INSTITUTIONAL REVIEW BOARD QUESTIONNAIRE FOR RESEARCHERS ON THE PROGRESS OF STUDIES APPROVED BY THE COMMITTEE / BOARD

Please draw a circle around 'Yes' or 'No'.
Where applicable, indicate in the box the number of cases involved.
*(Please write **NA** if the question is not applicable to this study.)*

Ethics committee proposal number: ....
Date approved by the committee: ....
Name of investigator: ....
Title of project: ....
....

Commencement of study
- Has the study started?   **Yes   No**
- If 'No', please explain:
                                                          (tick box)

    Funding not available   ☐   ☐
    Difficulties in recruitment   ☐   ☐
    Investigation of adverse events
      in other centres   ☐   ☐
    Other, please specify   ☐   ☐
....
....
- Has the study been abandoned?   **Yes   No**

• If so, please explain. ....
....
....

Completion of study

• Has the study been completed?   **Yes   No**

Protocol amendments

• Was it necessary to amend the protocol
  for this study?   **Yes   No**
• If so, by whom?:
                                                (tick box)
  Sponsor   ☐
  Researcher   ☐
  Other, please specify   ☐
• If yes, please briefly describe the amendments. ....
....
....

Recruitment

                                                (tick box)
• Original target number of subjects: ☐
• Number actually recruited: ☐
• Were there any difficulties in recruiting
  subjects to this study?   **Yes   No**
• If 'Yes', please explain the difficulties:
                                                (tick box)
  Tightness of inclusion/exclusion criteria   ☐
  Rarity of condition   ☐
  Unwilling to put up with discomfort   ☐
  Too time consuming for subject   ☐
  Difficulties with domestic arrangements   ☐
  Transport difficulties   ☐
  Other, please specify   ☐

Provision of information

• To whom was information about the project
  given? (Give numbers)
  Subject   ☐
  Relative/carer   ☐

Subject *and* relative/carer ☐
No one, please explain ☐

....

- How was information about the project given to
each subject or relative/carer? (Give numbers)

	subject	relative/carer
Verbally only	☐	☐
Written subject information sheet only	☐	☐
Verbal *and* written	☐	☐
Other, please specify	☐	☐

....

- Where did each subject or relative/carer receive
the information about the project? (Give numbers)

	subject	relative/carer
In hospital ward	☐	☐
At outpatient clinic	☐	☐
In family doctor surgery	☐	☐
At home, personal contact	☐	☐
At home, by post	☐	☐
Other, please specify		

....

- Time allowed between providing information
and requesting consent (hours):

subject	relative/carer
☐	☐

If variable, please explain

....

Obtaining consent

- Were any subjects unable to give informed
consent? **Yes   No**
- If yes, please explain the reasons for the inability.
(Give numbers)

Baby or infant ☐
Child unable to understand the nature of
the research ☐
Severity of illness ☐
Alzheimer's disease ☐
Intellectual disability ☐

Other severe mental illness ☐

Other, please specify ☐

- How was consent obtained? (Give numbers)

	subject	relative/carer
Verbal only	☐	☐
Written only	☐	☐
Verbal *and* Written	☐	☐
Consent not obtained	☐	☐
Other, please specify	☐	☐

....

If no consent obtained, please explain why not. ....

....

....

- Who obtained consent? (Give numbers)

	subject	relative/carer
Senior researcher	☐	☐
Other researcher	☐	☐
Doctor in charge of patient	☐	☐
Nursing staff	☐	☐
Other, please specify	☐	☐

Withdrawal of consent

- Did any patients/volunteers withdraw from the study?   **Yes**   **No**
- If any, please explain why they withdrew. (Give numbers)

Side-effects	☐
Discomfort	☐
Lack of efficacy	☐
Difficulties with domestic arrangements	☐
Transport difficulties	☐
No reason given	☐
Other, please specify	☐

....

- Who made the decision to withdraw? (Give numbers)

Subject	☐
Relative/carer	☐

Researcher ☐
Joint subject/researcher ☐
Other, please specify ☐

Adverse events

- Did any serious adverse events occur locally in
  this study? **Yes** **No**
- If, yes, how many serious adverse events occurred? ☐
- If applicable, how many serious adverse events
  occurred in all centres? ☐
- Please provide a summary of any new information
  that has arisen, since ethics committee approval,
  about risks associated with the study.

Outcome of research

- Did the study answer the research question that was
  being asked? **Yes** **No**
- If 'No', please explain why not:
  Study terminated owing to adverse events ☐
  Unable to recruit sufficient subjects ☐
  Other, please specify ☐

  ....

- Is a copy of the final report on the study available? **Yes** **No**
- If not, please explain the reasons:
  Study not yet complete ☐
  Report in preparation ☐
  Awaiting report from sponsor ☐
  Other, please specify ☐

  ....

- Has it been published? **Yes** **No**
- If so, please give the reference(s) ....

  ....

**Please attach a copy of the current patient information
sheet/consent form.**

Researcher's signature ....
Researcher's name (*in capitals*) ....
Date ....

► Further reading

The following are some key publications that may serve as a starting point for readers who wish to delve more deeply into the subject. For the complete reference, please refer to the main reference list.

Animal to human transplantation

An excellent review of the subject and the ethical issues raised by it, is to be found in the Nuffield Council on Bioethics Report (1996). In common with the other Nuffield reports a further reading list is provided.

Arrangements for compensation

The Association of the British Pharmaceutical Industry (ABPI), *Clinical Trial Compensation Guidelines* (ABPI 1991) is the key British document in this area. An interesting discussion of the whole question of compensation is provided by Guest (1997).

Clinical trials

The International Conference on Harmonisation (ICH) *Guideline for Good Clinical Practice*, for the United States, Europe and Japan, is essential reading (ICH 1996). The Association of the British Pharmaceutical Industry (ABPI) also produces a series of guidelines covering different aspects of clinical trials (see ABPI 1988 to 1995). They should be contacted for their latest updates. A classic paper on the subject of clinical trials is by Bradford Hill (1963).

For the latest drafts of other ICH reports and European Directives see under 'Some useful websites'.

The Commission of the European Communities, Directive 91/507/EEC, July 19 (1991) provides the legal basis for the *Good Clinical Practice for Trials on Medicinal Products in the European Community*.

Cloning

A consultation document entitled *Cloning Issues in Reproduction, Science and Medicine* was issued by the UK Human Genetics Advisory Commission (HGAC) and the Human Fertilisation and Embryo Authority in January 1998 (HGAC 1998).

Confidentiality

The Data Protection Act Guidelines (Data Protection Registrar, 1989) are essential reading for researchers in Britain whose research involves computerised databases.* The Royal College of Physicians' report (1994) on the ethical review of studies involving personal medical records and the recent Department of Health (1996a) guidelines on the protection and use of patient information will also be of interest.

Epidemiological studies

Readers are referred to the guidelines produced by the Council for International Organizations of Medical Sciences in collaboration with the World Health Organization (CIOMS/WHO 1991).

Evaluating risks and benefits

An introduction to the problem of trying to balance the two is provided by Evans (1993). Nicholson (1986) discusses risk in his book on research with children.

---

* The Act was revised in 1998 (for 1999 implementation) to cover some manual records.

Genetic research

For an introduction to the ethical issues surrounding genetic screening, readers are referred to the Nuffield Council on Bioethics (1993) report on the subject, to a recent book which discusses the issues surrounding genetic counselling (Clark 1994) and a report of the House of Commons Science and Technology Committee (1995).

Readers wishing to explore various sides of the argument may be interested in a series of papers in the *British Medical Journal*. For this example, this journal takes one genetically determined disease – hypertrophic cardiomyopathy – and discusses from several viewpoints the ethical issues surrounding genetic testing. (Davis 1995; Grigg 1995; Harper and Clarke 1995; Ryan et al. 1995).

For those interested in the implication of genetic testing for insurance, readers are referred to a paper by the UK Human Genetics Advisory Commission (1997).

Gene therapy

The Report of the Committee on the Ethics of Gene Therapy (Clothier 1992) provides a readable overview of the subject with important recommendations. Practical information on the type of gene therapy being attempted in the UK and elsewhere can be obtained from the annual reports of the Gene Therapy Advisory Committee.

Guidelines

The following are essential reading: the Declaration of Helsinki (reproduced in Appendix 1) and the guidelines produced by the Council for International Organizations of Medical Sciences in association with the World Health Organization (CIOMS/WHO 1993) and by the Royal College of Physicians (1996).

In the United States, a guidebook has been prepared by the Office for Protection from Research Risks, National Institutes of Health (1993) to assist institutional review board members and researchers in fulfilling their responsibilities for protecting the rights and welfare of human subjects as defined in the Department of Health and Human Services regulations entitled, *Protection of Human Subjects* (45 CFR, 46) and the Food and Drug Administration (FDA) Regulations (21 Code of Federal Regulations, parts 50 and 56). The FDA web site http://www.fda.gov/ also contains a wealth of information. These, plus the Belmont Report (1979), are essential reading for those interested in the ethical regulation of medical research in the United States.

A current *Catalogue of European Guidelines* can be obtained from the Medicines Control Agency, EuroDirect Publication Service, and explanatory leaflets on the Medicines Act 1968 and *Guidance on Applications for Clinical Trials Certificates and Clinical Trials Exemptions* can be obtained from the Medicines Control Agency, DHSS Medicines Division (see under 'Some Useful Addresses'). The first substantive UK documentation on the ethical aspects of research with human subjects was published by the Medical Research Council (1963).

Guidelines for specific types of study or patient groups are referenced in the text. The loose leaf manuals produced by Foster (1997) and by the Association of Independent Clinical Research Contractors (AICRC) at its excellent training conference for ethics committee members held annually in Cambridge, England, are convenient sources of many of these guidelines (see for example AICRC 1997).

Importance of informed consent

The rights and wrongs of not obtaining informed consent in two studies – the first relating to the kind of support offered to stroke victims (Dennis et al. 1997) and the second, the influence of HIV status on the outcome of patients admitted to intensive care (Bhagwanjee et al. 1997a) – were discussed at length in a series of recent articles in the British Medical Journal (Bhagwanjee et al 1997b; Dennis 1997; Kale 1997; McLean 1997; Seedat 1997; Smith 1997), and are recommended to readers interested in this issue. Of historical importance is the publication by Papworth (1967).

Journals

Several widely read medical journals, including the *British Medical Journal* and the *New England Journal of Medicine*, regularly carry papers and editorials on ethical issues relating to medical research. The short review articles of the *Bulletin of Medical Ethics* provide a convenient way of keeping up-to-date with developments in research ethics. *The Journal of Medical Ethics* is also a good source of discussion papers on the subject.

Medical ethics

For readers interested in exploring the philosophy underlying the ethical regulation of medical research and gaining an overview of medical ethics in general, the following books are suggested as an introduction:

> British Medical Association's Ethics, Science and Information Division (1993). *Medical Ethics Today: its Practice and Philosophy*.
> Campbell et al. (1997). *Medical Ethics*.
> Gillon (1986). *Philosophical Medical Ethics*.
> Mason and McCall Smith (1991). *Law and Medical Ethics*, 3rd edtn.

Of US historical interest, containing extensive reference literature on the subject prior to 1976 readers should refer to Humber and Almeder (1976).

Medical research ethics committees

Readers interested in the structure and functioning of research ethics committees in the UK can obtain further information from the Department of Health guidelines (DoH 1991, 1994) and their briefing pack for new members (DoH 1997a). The early survey of ethics committees by Neuberger (1992) will also be of interest as will the recent survey by Nicholson (1997a) on the extent to which committees are conforming to the 1991 Department of Health guidelines. A training video for insitutional review board members prepared by the US National Institutes of Health (NIH) and the Food and Drug Administration entitled *Protecting Human Subjects* (1986, reissued 1993) is available from the NIH (see under 'Some Useful Addresses, Department of Health and Human Services').

Placebos
Rothman and Michels (1994), Collier (1995) and De Deyn and D'Hooge (1996) provide an introduction to the debate on the ethics of using placebos.

Post-approval review
The Association of the British Pharmaceutical Industry (ABPI) has produced guidelines for the monitoring of clinical trials conducted by representatives of the sponsoring pharmaceutical company (ABPI 1994a). For a description of a pilot study regarding the post-approval monitoring of all kinds of studies by an ethics committee, readers are referred to the paper by Smith, Moore and Tunstall-Pedoe 1997.

Research on fetuses/unborn babies
The main official guidance on this issue continues to be the Polkinghorne Report (1989). For a discussion of the points for and against see *Human Embryo Research, Yes or No?* (CIBA 1986).

Research with healthy volunteers
The Royal College of Physicians (1986a) has produced guidelines as has the Association of the British Pharmaceutical Industry (1988).

Research on surplus blood and other tissue
Readers interested in the ethical and legal issues surrounding the use of human tissue are referred to the Nuffield Council on Bioethics (1995) report on the subject which also contains a useful list of references.

Vulnerable groups

For those interested in the ethics of research with children, relevant books on this subject include one from the UK by Nicholson (1986) and one from the USA edited by Grodin and Glantz (1994). Guidelines have also been issued by the British Paediatric Association (1992) and Medical Research Council (1991a), while for the involvement of children in pharmaceutical trials, the recent guideline produced by the European Agency for the Evaluation of Medicinal Products (1997) is a must.

The Alzheimer's Disease Society (1993) and the Royal College of Psychiatrists (1990) and Medical Research Council (1991b) in the UK have produced guidelines for patients with mental health problems, while the Office for Protection from Research Risks (OPRR) in the USA has produced guidelines regarding emergency research (OPRR1996).

The Association for Improvement in the Maternity Services, National Childbirth Trust and the Maternity Alliance (1997) has tackled the issue of maternity patients as a vulnerable group.

► Some useful websites

Association of the British Pharmaceutical Industry (ABPI)
http://www.abpi.org.uk/
Provides a list of members and links to their home pages.

British Medical Journal
http://www.bmj.com
Abstracts and full text of papers.

Bulletin of Medical Ethics
http://ourworld.compuserve.com/homepages/Bulletin_of_
    Medical_Ethics

Code of Federal Regulations
http://www.access.gpo.gov/nara/cfr/
The US regulations pertaining to the ethical regulation of medical
research can be obtained by going to the above site and searching for
keywords, including '45CFR46' and '21CFR50' and '21CFR56'.

Committee on Safety of Medicines (CSM)
http://www.open.gov.uk/mca/csmhome.htm
Contains information about the committee and its functions; gives
details of the Yellow Card System which includes a list of new drugs
for which all adverse reactions should be reported.

Committee for Proprietary Medicinal Products (CPMP)
http://www.eudra.org/emea.html
Copies of CPMP guidance papers, both adopted and draft, can be
obtained from this source, including the International Conference
on Harmonization good clinical practice guidelines.

Department of Health (England and Wales)
http://www.open.gov.uk/doh/dhhome.htm
Includes a list of health service guidelines which can be
downloaded.

European Agency for the Evaluation of Medicinal Products
http://www.eudra.org/emea.html
(i.e., same as CPMP site above).
Much of the statutory work on pharmaceutical products in the
European Union now falls to the European Medicines Evaluation
Agency (EMEA). Their site is a good starting point for more
information.

Food and Drug Administration (FDA)
http://www.fda.gov/
There is a particularly interesting set of papers entitled; 'IRB
Operations and Clinical Investigation Requirements' at
http://www.fda.gov/oc/oha/IRB/toc.html

Human Fertilisation and Embryology Authority (UK) (HFEA)
Can be accessed via the CCTA Government Information Service
website:
http://www.open.gov.uk
Search the index for HFEA.

Human Genetics Advisory Commission (UK)
http://www.dti.gov.uk/hgac
Includes consultation documents.

Institutional Review Board Guidebook, 1993
Office for Protection from Research Risks – NIH
http://www.nih.gov/grants/oprr/irb/inb_guidebook.htm

International Conference on Harmonisation
http:/www.ifpma.org/ich1.html
Managed by the International Federation of Pharmaceutical
Manufacturers Associations, this is the Secretariat for the
International Conference on Harmonization (ICH). From here you can
discover the current situation with all ICH guidelines and download
full text versions.

Journal of the American Medical Association
Access via the American Medical Association web site:
http://www.ama-assn.org
Abstracts of papers.

Journal of Medical Ethics
http://www.jmedethics.com
Index and reprint ordering information.

Medicines Control Agency
http://www.open.gov.uk/mca/mcahome.htm
Currently (i.e. December 1998) details of the Agency's structure and
function are available but soon the website is to be expanded to give
details of all aspects of medicines regulation in the UK.

Medical Devices Agency (UK)
http://www.medical-devices.gov.uk

Medical Research Council (UK)
http://www.mrc.ac.uk

Royal College of Physicians of London
http://www.rcplondon.ac.uk/

Scottish Office
http://www.Scotland.gov.uk
For full text Scottish Office publications

US Health and Human Services Department
http://www.hhs.gov/

World Health Organization (WHO)
http://www.who.ch/

WHO publications
http://www.who.ch/pll/dsa/cat98/zcon.htm
Abstracts and ordering information.

► Some useful addresses

Alzheimer's Disease Society
Gordon House
10 Greencoat Place
London SW1P 1PH
UK

Association of the British
Pharmaceutical Industry
12 Whitehall
London SW1A 2DY
UK
(For copies of the Guidelines)

Association of Independent Clinical
Research Contractors
PO Box 1055
Oadby
Leicester LE2 4XZ
UK

British Paediatric Association
5 St Andrew's Place
Regents Park
London NW1 4LB
UK
Tel: 0171 486 6151

British Psychological Society
St Andrews House
48 Princess Road East
Leicester LE1 7DR
UK

British Sociological Society
Unit 3G
Mountjoy Research Centre
Stockton Road
Durham DH1 3UR
UK

Centre for Medical Law and Ethics
Kings College
Strand
London WC2R 2LS
UK

Council for International
Organization of Medical Sciences
(CIOMS)
c/o World Health Organization
Avenue Appia
1211 Geneva 27
Switzerland
Tel: (00 41 22) 791 2111
Fax: (00 41 22) 791 0746

Council of Europe
Editions du Conseil de l'Europe
F-67075 Strasbourg Cedex
France

Department of Health
PO Box 410
Wetherby LS23 7LL
UK
(For Health Service guidelines and
'Briefing Pack for LREC Members')

Department of Health and Human
Services
Public Health Service
National Institutes of Health
Office for Protection from Research
    Risks
6100 Executive Blvd
Suite 3B01 MSC 7507
Rockville
MD 20892-7507
USA
(For copy of training video 'Protecting
Human Subjects')

DHSS Medicines Division (Medicines
Control Agency)
Clinical Trials Exemption Scheme
Room 1117
Market Towers
1 Nine Elms Lane
London SW8 5NQ
UK

European Forum for Clinical Practice
Schoolbergenstraat 47
B-3030 Kessel-Lo (Leuven)
Belgium

Human Fertilisation and Embryology
Authority
Paxton House
30 Artillery Lane
London E1 7LS
UK

IFPMA
30 rue de St Jean
PO Box 9
1211 Geneva 18
Switzerland
(For International Conference on
Harmonisation 'Guideline for Good
Clinical Practice')

Medical Research Council
20 Park Crescent
London W1N 4AL
UK

Medicines Control Agency
Eurodirect Publications Office
Room 1205
Market Towers (Information Centre)
1 Nine Elms Lane
London SW8 5NQ
UK
(For CPMP publications)

Mental Health Act Commission
Maid Marian House
56 Hounds Gate
Nottingham NG1 6BG
UK

Multicentre Research Ethics
Committee Scotland
Deaconess House
148 Pleasance
Edinburgh EH8 9RS
UK

National Union of Students
Nelson Mandela House
461 Holloway Road
London N7 6LJ
UK
(For guidance to students participating
in medical research)

NHS Management Executive
St Andrews House
Edinburgh EH1 3DG
UK

Nuffield Council on Bioethics
28 Bedford Square
London WC1B 3EG
UK

Office of the Data Protection Registrar
Springfield House
Water Lane
Wilmslow
Cheshire SK9 5AX
UK

Royal College of General Practitioners
14 Princes Gate
Hyde Park
London SW7 1PU
UK

Royal College of Nursing
20 Cavendish Square
London W1M 0AB
UK

Royal College of Physicians
11 St Andrews Place
London NW1 4LE
UK

Royal College of Psychiatrists
17 Belgrave Square
London SW1X 8PG
UK

Royal Society of Medicine Services Ltd
1 Wimpole Street
London W1M 8AE
UK

Superintendent of Documents
PO Box 371954
Pittsburgh
PA 15250-795
USA
*(For Office for Protection from Research
Risks publications)*

► Bibliography

Advisors to the President of the European Commission on the Ethical
Implications of Biotechnology (1997). Ethical aspects of cloning
techniques. *Journal of Medical Ethics*, **23**, 349–52.

Advisory Group on the Ethics of Xenotransplantation (1997). *Animal Tissue
into Humans*. London:HMSO.

Alberti, K.G.M.M. (1995). Local research ethics committees. *British Medical
Journal*, **311**, 639–40.

Allan, J. (1997). Silk purse or sow's ear. *Nature Medicine*, **3**, 275–6.

Allen, M.E. (Ed.) (1991). *Good Clinical Practice in Europe, Investigator's
Handbook*. Romford: Rostrum Publications.

Alzheimer's Disease Society (1993). *Volunteering for Research into Dementia*.
London: Alzheimer's Disease Society.

Amdur, R.J. and Biddie, C. (1997). Institutional review board approval and
publication of human research results. *Journal of the American Medical
Association*, **277**, 909–14.

Angell, M. (1997). Ethics of clinical research in the third world. *New
England Journal of Medicine*, **337**, 847–9.

Anon. (1996a). Unilever's Central Ethical Compliance group. *Bulletin of
Medical Ethics*, No. 122, 14.

Anon. (1996b). Reinventing the research ethics board in Canada. *Bulletin of
Medical Ethics*, No. 122, 15–17.

Anon. (1997a). Research involving detained patients: Mental Health Act
Commission *Bulletin of Medical Ethics*, no. 129, 8–11.

Anon. (1997b). Cloning animals and human beings: the European
Parliament. *Bulletin of Medical Ethics*, no. 128, 10–11.

Anon. (1997c). Multi-centre research ethics committees. *Bulletin of Medical
Ethics*, no. 127, 3–6.

Aspinal, R.L. and Goodman, N.W. (1995). Denial of effective treatment and poor quality of clinical information in placebo controlled trials of ondansetron for postoperative nausea and vomiting: a review of published trials. *British Medical Journal*, **311**, 844–6.

Association of the British Pharmaceutical Industry (1990a). *Guidelines for Research Ethics Committees Considering Studies Conducted in Healthy Volunteers by Pharmaceutical Companies*. London: Association of the British Pharmaceutical Industry.

Association of the British Pharmaceutical Industry (1990b). *Guidelines for Medical Experiments in Non-Patient Human Volunteers. (March 1988, with amendments May 1990)*. London: Association of the British Pharmaceutical Industry.

Association of the British Pharmaceutical Industry (1991). *Clinical Trial Compensation Guidelines*. London: Association of the British Pharmaceutical Industry.

Association of the British Pharmaceutical Industry (1992).*Good Clinical (Research) Practice*. London: Association of the British Pharmaceutical Industry.

Association of the British Pharmaceutical Industry (1993).*Guidelines for Phase IV Clinical Trials*. London: Association of the British Pharmaceutical Industry.

Association of the British Pharmaceutical Industry (1994a).*Guidelines on the Conduct of Investigator Site Audits*. London: Association of the British Pharmaceutical Industry.

Association of the British Pharmaceutical Industry (1994b). *Relationships between the medical profession and the pharmaceutical industry*. London: Association of the British Pharmaceutical Industry.

Association of the British Pharmaceutical Industry (1994c). *Guidelines for Company-Sponsored Safety Assessment of Marketed Medicines (SAMM)*. London: Association of the British Pharmaceutical Industry.

Association of the British Pharmaceutical Industry (1995). *Good Clinical Trial Practice for Investigators Taking Part in Non-industry Sponsored Research*. London: Association of the British Pharmaceutical Industry.

Association of the British Pharmaceutical Industry et al. (1988). Guideline on post-marketing surveillance. *British Medical Journal*, **296**, 399–400.

Association of the British Pharmaceutical Industry et al. (1993). *Guideline for company sponsored safety assessment of marketed products*. London: Department of Health.

Association for Improvement in the Maternity Services, National Childbirth Trust and the Maternity Alliance (AIMS) (1997). A charter for ethical research in maternity care. *Bulletin of Medical Ethics,* **130,** 8–11.

Association of Independent Clinical Research Contractors (1992). *Guidelines for Research Ethics Committees.* London: Association of Independent Clinical Research Contractors.

Association of Independent Clinical Research Contractors (1997). *Ethical Review of Clinical Research: A Training Conference for Ethics Committee Members, Delegates Folder,* London: Association of Independent Clinical Research Contractors.

Beecher, H.K. (1966) Ethics and Clinical Research. *New England Journal of Medicine,* **274,** 1354–60.

Belmont Report (1979). *Ethical Principles and Guidelines for the Protection of Human Research Subjects.* The National Commission for the Protection of Human Subjects of Biomedical and Behavioral Research. Federal Report Document 79-12065, Washington.

Bendall, C.H. (1994). *Standard Operating Procedures for Local Research Ethics Committees. Comments and examples.* London: McKenna & Co.

Bhagwanjee, S., Muckart, D.J.J., Jeena, P.M. and Moodley, P. (1997a). Does HIV status influence the outcome of patients admitted to a surgical intensive care unit? A prospective double blind study. *British Medical Journal,* **314,** 1077–82.

Bhagwanjee, S., Muckart, D.J.J., Jeena, P.M. and Moodley, P. (1997b). Commentary: why we did not seek informed consent before testing patients for HIV. *British Medical Journal,* **314,** 1082–3.

Bradford Hill, A. (1963). Medical ethics and controlled trials. *British Medical Journal,* 1, 1043–9.

British Medical Association's Ethics, Science and Information Division (1993). *Medical Ethics Today; its Practice and Philosophy.* London: BMJ Publishing Group.

British Paediatric Association (1992). *Ethics Advisory Committee Guidelines for the Ethical Conduct of Medical Research involving Children.* London: British Paediatric Association.

British Psychological Society (1993). Ethical principles for conducting research with human participants. *The Psychologist* **6,** 6–12.

British Sociological Society (1993). *Statement of Ethical Practice.* Durham: British Sociological Society.

Brown, W.A. (1994). Placebo as a treatment for depression. *Neuropsychopharmacology,* **10,** 265–9.

Bulfield, G. (1998). Quoted in: 'Doctors call for human cloning ban'. *The Times* (January 8), pp. 1–2. London.

Bulmer, M. (Ed.) (1982). *Social Research Ethics*. London: The Macmillan Press.

Campbell, A., Charlesworth, M., Gillet, G. and Jones, G. (1997). *Medical Ethics*. Auckland, New Zealand: Oxford University Press.

21 CFR (Code of Federal Regulations dealing with clinical studies, including parts 50 and 56 concerning Informed Consent and IRB Regulations). The Food and Drug Administration regulations. http://www.fda.gov

45 CFR (Code of Federal Regulations, Title 45) (1991), *Part 46 Protection of Human Subjects*. Washington: Department of Health and Human Services and Office for Protection from Research Risks.

Champey, Y., Levine, R.J. and Lietman, P.S. (1989). *Development of New Medicines: Ethical Questions*. Proceedings of a symposium sponsored by Fondation Rhone-Poulenc Sante, held in Paris, 2 December 1988. London: Royal Society of Medicine Services Ltd.

CIBA Foundation (1986). Human Embryology Research, Yes or No? London: Tavistock Publications.

CIOMS/WHO (1991). *International Guidelines for Ethical Review of Epidemiological Studies*. Geneva: Council for International Organisations of Medical Sciences/World Health Organisation.

CIOMS/WHO (1993). *International Ethical Guidelines for Biomedical Research Involving Human Subjects. (Revised version of the 1982 Proposed Guidelines for Biomedical Research Involving Human Subjects). CIOMS in collaboration with the World Health Organisation*. Geneva: Council for International Organisations of Medical Sciences/World Health Organisation.

Clark, A. (Ed.) (1994). *Genetic Counselling; Practice and Principles*. London: Routledge.

Clothier, C.B. (Chairman) (1992). *Report of the Committee on the Ethics of Gene Therapy*. Cm. 1788. London: HMSO.

Collier, J. (1995). Confusion over the use of placebos in clinical trials. Better guidelines needed. *British Medical Journal*, **311**, 821–2.

Commission of the European Communities (1989). *The Rules Governing Medicinal Products in the European Community*, Vol.1. Catalogue No. CB-55-89-706-EN-C, (ISBN 92-825-9563-3).

Commission of the European Communities (1990). *Good Clinical Practice for Trials on Medicinal Products in the European Community*. 111/3976/88-EN [approved July 1990, effective July 1991]. Published in: *Pharmacology and Toxicology* (1990), **67**, 361–72.

Committee for Proprietary Medicinal Products (CPMP) Working Party on

Efficacy of Medicinal Products in the European Community (1990). *Notes for Guidance: Good Clinical Practice for Trials on Medicinal Products in the European Community*. CPMP 111/3976/88-EN. Strasbourg: Office for Official Publications of the European Communities.

Committee for Proprietary Medicinal Products (CPMP) European Agency for the Evaluation of Medicinal Products, Human Medicines Evaluation Unit (1997). *Note for Guidance on Clinical Investigation of Medicinal Products in Children*. MCA EuroDirect Publication No. CPMP EWP/462/95. London: Medical Control Agency.

Council of Europe (1997). *Convention for the Protection of Human Rights and Dignity of the Human Being with regard to the Application of Biology and Medicine*. Oviedo, 4.IV. European Treaty Series /164. Strasbourg: Editions du Conseil de l'Europe.

Cox, C. and Macpherson, C.N.L. (1996). Modified informed consent in a viral seroprevalence study in the Caribbean. *Bioethics*, **10**, 222–32.

Daniel, C. (1997). Locking sick out in the cold. *New Statesman* (21 February), pp. 22–3.

Data Protection Registrar (1989). *The Data Protection Act Guidelines*. Wilmslow: Office of the Data Protection Registrar.

Davis, J. (1995). Ethical issues. *British Medical Journal*, **310**, 858.

Deacon, T. (1997). Histological evidence of fetal pig neural cell survival after transplantation into a patient with Parkinson's disease. *Nature Medicine*, **3**, 350–3.

De Deyn, P.P. and D'Hooge, R. (1996). Placebos in clinical practice and research. *Journal of Medical Ethics*, **22**, 140–6.

Dennis, M. (1997). Why we didn't ask patients for their consent. *British Medical Journal*, **314**, 1077.

Dennis, M., O'Rourke, S., Slattery, J., Staniforth, T., and Warlow, C. (1997). Evolution of a stroke family care worker: results of a randomised controlled trial. *British Medical Journal*, **314**, 1071–7.

Department of Health (1991). *Local Research Ethics Committees*. HSG (91) 5. London: Department of Health.

Department of Health (1994). *Standards for Local Research Ethics Committees A Framework for Ethical Review*. London: NHS Training Division.

Department of Health (1996a). *The Protection and Use of Patient Information*. HSG(96)18, LASSL(96). London: Department of Health.

Department of Health (1996b). *NHS Indemnity: Arrangements for Handling Clinical Negligence Claims Against NHS Staff. HSG(96)48*. London: Department of Health.

Department of Health (1997a). *Briefing Pack for LREC Members*. London: Department of Health.

Department of Health (1997b). *Ethics Committee Review of Multi-centre Research: Establishment of Multi-centre Research Ethics Committees.* HSG(97)23. London: Department of Health, PO Box 410, Wetherby, LS23 7LL, England.

Department of Health/ The Scottish Office (1997). *Multi-centre Research Ethics Committee for Scotland.* NHS MEL (1997) 8. Edinburgh: NHS Management Executive.

Department of Health (1998). *Letter to all Research Ethics Committee Chairmen from A. J. M. Palmer.* The Scottish Office, NHS Management Executive, 21 May.

Dyer, C. (1997). Consultant struck off over research fraud. *British Medical Journal,* **315**, 205.

European Forum for Good Clinical Practice (1997). *Guidelines and Recommendations for European Ethics Committees.* Kessel-Lo: European Forum for Clinical Practice. Schoolbergenstraat 47, B-3010 Kessel-Lo (Leuven), Belgium.

Evans, M. (1993). Evaluating risks and benefits. In *Ethical Review of Clinical Research, A Training Conference for Ethics Committee Members, Delegates Folder (1997).* London: The Association of Independent Clinical Research Contractors.

Evans, D. and Evans, M. (1996). *A Decent Proposal.* Chichester: John Wiley & Sons Ltd.

Faden, R (1996). The Advisory Committee on Human Radiation Experiments. *Hastings Centre Report.* **26** (5), 5–10.

Foster, C.G. (Ed.) (1997). *Manual for Research Ethics Committees,* 5th edn. London: Centre for Medical Law and Ethics.

Fulford, K.W.M. and Howse, K. (1993). Ethics of research with psychiatric patients: principles, problems and the primary responsibility of researchers. *Journal of Medical Ethics,* **19**, 85–91.

Gene Therapy Advisory Committee (1994). *Guidance on Making Proposals to Conduct Gene Therapy Research on Human Subjects.* London: Department of Health.

Gene Therapy Advisory Committee (1995). *First Annual Report November 1993 to December 1994.* London: Department of Health.

Gene Therapy Advisory Committee (1996). *Second Annual Report 1995.* London: Department of Health.

Gentzkow, G.D., Iwasaki S.D., Hershon K.S., Mengel M., Prendergast J.J.,

Ricotta J.J., Steed D.P. and Lipkin S. (1996). Use of Dermagraft, a cultured human dermis, to treat diabetic foot ulcers. *Diabetic Care*, **8**, 350–4.

Gillon, R. (1986). *Philosophical Medical Ethics*. London: John Wiley & Sons Ltd.

Goldberg, D. (1981). *General Health Questionnaire – 28*. Windsor: NFER-NELSON Publishing Company.

Goodman, N.W. and Edwards, M.B. (1997). *Medical Writing: A Prescription for Clarity*. Cambridge: Cambridge University Press.

Grigg, L. (1995). Knowledge of risk allows adaptation. *British Medical Journal*, **310**, 859.

Grodin, M.A. and Glantz, L.H. (Eds.) (1994). *Children as Research Subjects: Science Ethics and Law*. Oxford: Oxford University Press.

Grubb, A (1997). The law relating to consent. In *Manual for Research Ethics Committees*, 5th edn. ed. C.G. Foster, pp. 11–17. London: Centre for Medical Law and Ethics.

Guest, S. (1997). Compensation for subjects of medical research: the moral rights of patients and the power of research ethics committees. *Journal of Medical Ethics*, **23**, 181–5.

Harper, P.S. (1993). Research samples from families with genetic diseases: a proposed code of conduct. *British Medical Journal*, **306**, 1391–4.

Harper, P.S. and Clarke, A. (1995). Testing may be unhelpful. *British Medical Journal*, **310**, 857–8.

House of Commons Science and Technology Committee (1995). *Human Genetics: the Science and the Consequences*. London: HMSO.

Human Fertilisation and Embryology Authority (1995). *Code of Practice*. London: Human Fertilisation and Embryology Authority.

Human Genetics Advisory Commission (1997). *The Implications of Genetic Testing for Insurance*. http://www.dti.gov.uk/hgac/papers.

Human Genetics Advisory Commission (1998). *Cloning Issues in Reproduction, Science and Medicine*. http://www.dti.gov.uk/hgac/papers.

Humber, J.M. and Almeder, R.F. (Eds.) (1976). New guidelines on research with human subjects. In *Biomedical Ethics and the Law*, pp. 277–304. New York: Plenum Press.

International Conference on Harmonisation, (ICH) (1993). *Clinical Safety Data Management- definitions and standards for expedited reporting* (111/3375/93/Final). Geneva: IFPMA.

International Conference on Harmonisation of Technical Requirements for Registration of Pharmaceuticals for Human Use. (ICH) (1996). *Guideline for Good Clinical Practice*. Geneva: IFPMA.

Instituto di Bioetica (1996). Against experimentation on human embryos. Statement translated in *Bulletin of Medical Ethics*, **122**, 9–11.

Kahn, A. (1997). Clone mammals, clone man? *Nature,* **386**, 119.

Kale, R. (1997). Commentary: failing to seek patients' consent to research is always wrong. *British Medical Journal*, **314**, 1081–2.

La Puma, J., Stocking, C.B., Rhoades, W.D. and Darling, C.M. (1995). Financial ties as part of informed consent to postmarketing research. *British Medical Journal*, **310**, 1660–3.

Mason, J.K. and McCall Smith, R.A. (1991) *Law and Medical Ethics*, 3rd edn. London: Butterworths.

McLean, S. (1997). No consent means not treating the patient with respect. *British Medical Journal*, **314**, 1076.

Medical Research Council (1963). Responsibility in investigations on human subjects. *MRC Annual Report for 1962–63*. London: Medical Research Council.

Medical Research Council (1991a). *The Ethical Conduct of Research on Children*. London: Medical Research Council.

Medical Research Council (1991b). *The Ethical Conduct of Research on the Mentally Incapacitated*. London: Medical Research Council.

Medical Research Council (1991c). *The Ethical Conduct of AIDS Vaccine Trials*. London: Medical Research Council.

Medical Research Council (1992a). *Responsibility in Investigations on Human Participants and Material and on Personal Information*. London: Medical Research Council.

Medical Research Council (1992b). New MRC guidance on research ethics. *Bulletin of Medical Ethics*, **84**, 18–23. [an update of the 1963 guidance].

Medical Research Council (1994). *Responsibility in the Use of Personal Medical Information for Research: Principles and Guide for Practice*. London: Medical Research Council.

Mental Health Act Commission (1997). *Research Involving Detained Patients. Position paper 1, January 1997*. Nottingham: Mental Health Act Commission.

Middle, C., Johnson, A., Petty, T., Sims, L. and Macfarlane, A. (1995). Ethics approval for a national postal survey: recent experience. *British Medical Journal*, **311**, 659–60.

Morgan, D. and Lee, R.G.(Eds.) (1990). In *Blackstone's Guide to the Human*

Fertilisation and Embryology Act 1990, pp. 186–225. London: Blackstone Press.

Multicentre Research Ethics Committee for Scotland (1997). *Multicentre Research Ethics Committee: Notes For Researchers*. Edinburgh: MREC Scotland.

National Bioethics Advisory Commission (1997). Cloning human beings. *Bulletin of Medical Ethics*, **131**, 8–10.

National Institutes of Health (1989). *Points to Consider in the Design and Submission of Human Somatic Cell Gene Therapy Protocols*. Federal Register 54, 36698-36703, Washington.

National Radiological Protection Board (1988). *Guidance Notes for the Protection of Persons Against Ionising Radiation Arising from Medical and Dental Use*. London: HMSO.

National Union of Students [no date available]. *Guidelines for Students Participating in Medical Experiments*. London: National Union of Students.

Neuberger J. (1992). *Ethics and Health Care*. King's Fund Institute Research Report. London: King's Fund.

Nicholson, R. H. (1986) *Medical Research with Children: Ethics, Law and Practice*. Oxford: Oxford University Press.

Nicholson, R.H. (1997a) What do they get up to? LREC Annual Reports. *Bulletin of Medical Ethics* **129**, 13–24.

Nicholson, R.H. (1997b) Ethics and the use of ionising radiation in research on humans. *Bulletin of Medical Ethics*, **132**, 13–24.

Nuffield Council on Bioethics (1993). *Genetic Screening, Ethical Issues*. London: Nuffield Council on Bioethics.

Nuffield Council on Bioethics (1995). *Human Tissue, Ethical and Legal Issues*. London: Nuffield Council on Bioethics.

Nuffield Council on Bioethics (1996). *Animal-to-Human Transplants, the Ethics of Xenotransplantation*. London: Nuffield Council on Bioethics.

Nuremberg Code (1946). In *Permissible Medical Experiments, Trials of War Criminals before the Nuremberg Military Tribunals under Control Council Law No 10: Nuremberg October 1946–April 1949*, vol. 2, pp.181–2. Washington: US Government Printing Office.

Office for Protection from Research Risks, Department of Health and Human Services, National Institutes of Health (1984). *AIDS Guidance December 26. Guidance for Institutional Review Boards for AIDS Studies*. Bethesda: National Institutes of Health.

Office for Protection from Research Risks (1993). *Protecting Human Research Subjects. Institutional Review Board Guidebook*. Bethesda: Department of Health and Human Services.

Office for Protection from Research Risks (1995). *Continuing Review-Institutional and Institutional Review Board Responsibilities*. OPRR Reports Number 95-01, January 10. Rockville: National Institutes of Health.

Office for Protection from Research Risks (1996). *Informed Consent Requirements in Emergency Research*. OPRR Reports Number 97-01, October 31. Rockville: National Institutes of Health. [UK source: Bulletin of Medical Ethics (1997), **132** , 9–11.]

Office for Protection from Research Risks (1997). *Expedited Review of Certain Research*. OPRR Reports Number 97-02, February 20. Rockville: National Institutes of Health.

Olde-Rikkert, M.G.M., Bercken van den, J.H.L., Have ten, H.A.M.J. and Hoefnagels, W.H.L. (1997). *Journal of Medical Ethics*, **23**, 271–6.

Pappworth, M.H. (1967). *Human Guinea Pigs, Experimentation on Man*. London: Routledge & Kegan Paul.

Patience, C., Takeuchi, Y. and Weiss, R.A. (1997). Infection of human cells by an endogenous retrovirus of pig. *Nature Medicine*, **3**, 282–6.

Polkinghorne, J. and Members of the Committee. (1989). *Review of the Guidance on the Research Use of Foetuses and Foetal Material (The Polkinghorne Report). Presented to Parliament, Cm 762*. London: HMSO.

Rothman, K.I. and Michels, K.B. (1994). The continuing unethical use of placebo controls. *New England Journal of Medicine*, **331**, 394–8.

Royal College of General Practitioners, Clinical Research Ethics Committee (1995). *Some Guidelines for Applicants for Ethical Approval for Research Involving Patients in General Practice*. London: Royal College of General Practitioners.

Royal College of Nursing (1993). *Ethics Related to Research in Nursing*. Harrow: Scutari Publications.

Royal College of Physicians (1986a). *Research on Healthy Volunteers*. Report of a Working Party. London: Royal College of Physicians.

Royal College of Physicians (1986b). The relationship between physicians and the pharmaceutical industry. *Journal of the Royal College of Physicians, London*, **20**.

Royal College of Physicians. (1990a). *Guidelines on the Practice of Ethics Committees in Medical Research Involving Human Subjects*, 2nd edn. London: The Royal College of Physicians.

Royal College of Physicians (1990b). *Research Involving Patients.* London: The Royal College of Physicians.

Royal College of Physicians (1994). Independent ethical review of studies involving personal medical records. Report of a working group. *Journal of the Royal College of Physicians, London,* **28**, 429–43.

Royal College of Physicians (1996). *Guidelines on the Practice of Ethics Committees in Medical Research Involving Human Subjects,* 3rd edn. London: The Royal College of Physicians.

Royal College of Psychiatrists (1990). Guidelines for research ethics committees on psychiatric research involving human subjects. *Psychiatric Bulletin,* **14**, 48–61.

Ryan, M.P., French, J., Al-Mahdawi, S., Nihoyannopoulos, P., Cleland, J.G.F. and Oakley, C.M. (1995). Genetic testing for familial hypertrophic cardiomyopathy in newborn infants. *British Medical Journal,* **310**, 856–7.

Savulescu, J., Chalmers, I. and Blunt, J (1996). Are research ethics committees behaving unethically? Some suggestions for improving performance and accountability. *British Medical Journal,* **313**, 1390–3.

Scottish Office, Home and Health Department (1992). *Local Research Ethics Committees.* Edinburgh: The Scottish Office.

Scottish Office (1997). *The Establishment of a Multi-centre Research Ethics Committee for Scotland.* NHS MEL (1997)8. Edinburgh: Scottish Office.

Seedat, Y.K. (1997). Commentary: no simple and absolute ethical rule exists for every conceivable situation. *British Medical Journal,* **314**, 1083–4.

Sheriff's Report (1997). Fatal accident enquiry; death during research. *Bulletin of Medical Ethics,* **130**, 22–4.

Shimm, D.S. and Spece, R.G. (1991). Industry reimbursement for entering patients into clinical trials: legal and ethical issues. *Annals of Internal Medicine,* **115**, 148–51.

Silverman, W.A. and Altman, D. (1996). Patient's preferences and randomised trials. *Lancet,* **347**, 171–2.

Smith, R. (1995). Publishing information about patients. *British Medical Journal,* **311**, 1240–1.

Smith, R. (1996). Time to face up to research misconduct. *British Medical Journal,* **312**, 789–90.

Smith, R. (1997). Informed consent: the intricacies. *British Medical Journal,* **314**, 1059–60.

Smith, T., Moore, E.J.H. and Tunstall-Pedoe, H. (1997). Review by a local medical research ethics committee of the conduct of approved research projects, by examination of patient's case notes, consent forms, and research records and by interview. *British Medical Journal*, **314**, 1588–90.

Tobias, J.S. and Souhami, R.L. (1993). Fully informed consent may be needlessly cruel. *British Medical Journal*, **307**, 1199–201.

Tunstall-Pedoe, H. (1995). Local committees have strengths too. *British Medical Journal*, **311**, 1570–1.

Warnock, M. (1984). *Report of the Committee of Inquiry into Human Fertilisation and Embryology*. Department of Health and Social Security, Cmd 9314. London: HMSO.

Weijer, C., Shapiro, S., Fuks, A., Glass, K.C. and Strutkowska, M. (1995). Monitoring clinical research: an obligation unfulfilled. *Canadian Medical Association Journal*, **152**, 1973–80.

Weiss, R.B., Vogelzang, N.J., Peterson, B.A. et al. (1993). A successful system of scientific data audits for clinical trials. *Journal of the American Medical Association*, **270**, 459–64.

Wells, F. (1996). Recent developments. In *Fraud and Misconduct in Medical Research* ed. S. Lock and F. Wells, London: BMJ Publishing Group.

Wells, F. and Blunt, J. (1997). The role of LRECs in the prevention of fraud. *Bulletin of Medical Ethics*, **131**, 2.

Wiffen, P. and Reynolds, J. (1997). *Guidance on aspects of medicines research*. In *Manual for Research Ethics Committees*, 5th edn. ed. C.G. Foster, London: Centre for Medical Law and Ethics.

Wilmut, I, Schnleke, A.E., McWhir, J. et al. (1997). Viable offspring derived from fetal and adult mammalian cells. *Nature*, **385**, 810–13.

Winston, R. (1997). The promise of cloning for human medicine. *British Medical Journal*, **314**, 913–14

World Medical Association (1993). Declaration of Geneva 1947, amended by the 22nd World Medical Assembly, Sydney, Australia in August 1968 and the 35th World Medical Assembly, Venice, Italy, in October 1983. Reproduced in *Medical Ethics Today, Its Practice and Philosophy*, BMA Ethics, Science and Information Division et al. (1993), pp. 327–9. London: BMJ Publishing Group.

World Medical Association (1995). Declaration of Lisbon on the Rights of the Patient, as revised in Bali, Indonesia, September 1995. *Bulletin of Medical Ethics*, (1996), **14**, 8–10.

World Medical Association (1996). *World Medical Association Declaration of Helsinki: Recommendations Guiding Physicians in Biomedical Research Involving Human Subjects*. Adopted by the 18th World Medical Assembly,

Helsinki, Finland, June 1964. Amended by the 29th World Medical Assembly, Tokyo, Japan, October 1975; 35th World Medical Assembly, Venice, Italy, October 1983; 41st World Medical Assembly, Hong Kong, September 1989 and the 48th General Assembly, Somerset West, Republic of South Africa, October 1996. Reproduced in *Journal of the American Medical Association*, **277**, 925–6.

Yeung, M., O'Connor, A., Parry, D.T., and Cochrane, G.M. (1994). Compliance with prescribed drug therapy in asthma. *Respiratory Medicine*, **88**, 31–5.

► Index